Fitness AEROBICS

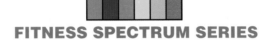

FITNESS SPECTRUM SERIES

Lynne Brick

Brick Bodies Fitness Services, Inc.

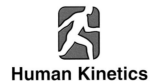

Human Kinetics

Library of Congress Cataloging-in-Publication Data

Brick, Lynne G., 1955-
    Fitness aerobics / Lynne G. Brick.
        p.   cm. -- (Fitness spectrum series)
    ISBN 0-87322-471-X
    1. Aerobic exercises.   I. Title.   II. Series.
    RA781.15.B75   1996   95-49231
    613.7'1--dc20   CIP

ISBN: 0-87322-471-X

Copyright © 1996 by Human Kinetics Publishers, Inc.

Developmental Editor: Marni Basic; **Assistant Editors:** Susan Moore and Julie Marx Ohnemus; **Editorial Assistants:** Jennifer J. Hemphill and Amy Carnes; **Copyeditor:** Holly Gilly; **Proofreader:** Karen Bojda; **Typesetting and Layout:** Ruby Zimmerman and Stuart Cartwright; **Text Designer:** Keith Blomberg; **Cover Designer:** Jack Davis; **Cover Photographer:** Ray Malace; **Photo Editor:** Boyd LaFoon; **Illustrators:** Keith Blomberg and Studio 2-D

Human Kinetics books are available at special discounts for bulk purchase. Special editions or book excerpts can also be created to specification. For details, contact the Special Sales Manager at Human Kinetics.

Printed in Hong Kong   10 9 8 7 6 5 4 3 2 1

Human Kinetics

Web site: http://www.humankinetics.com

United States: Human Kinetics, P.O. Box 5076, Champaign, IL 61825-5076
1-800-747-4457
e-mail: humank@hkusa.com

Canada: Human Kinetics, Box 24040, Windsor, ON N8Y 4Y9
1-800-465-7301 (in Canada only)
e-mail: humank@hkcanada.com

Europe: Human Kinetics, P.O. Box IW14, Leeds LS16 6TR, United Kingdom
(44) 1132 781708
e-mail: humank@hkeurope.com

Australia: Human Kinetics, 57A Price Avenue, Lower Mitcham, South Australia 5062
(08) 277 1555
e-mail: humank@hkaustralia.com

New Zealand: Human Kinetics, P.O. Box 105-231, Auckland 1
(09) 523 3462
e-mail: humank@hknewz.com

To my husband, Victor, our daughter Vicki, and our son Jonathan, who provide me with endless motivation, inspiration, support, and love.

Contents

Acknowledgments vi

Part I Preparing for Aerobics 1

 Chapter 1 Aerobics and Fitness 3
 Chapter 2 Getting Equipped 8
 Chapter 3 Checking Your Aerobic Fitness 16
 Chapter 4 Aerobics the Right Way 23
 Chapter 5 Warming Up and Cooling Down 40

Part II Aerobics Workout Zones 51

 Chapter 6 Green Zone 56
 Chapter 7 Blue Zone 63
 Chapter 8 Purple Zone 72
 Chapter 9 Yellow Zone 84
 Chapter 10 Orange Zone 101
 Chapter 11 Red Zone 116

Part III Training by the Workout Zones 131

 Chapter 12 Setting Up Your Program 133
 Chapter 13 Sample Aerobics Programs 138
 Chapter 14 Charting Your Progress 143

Appendix A Aerobics Moves 149

Appendix B Aerobics Music 167

About the Author 169

Acknowledgments

I thank the people (and organizations) who have helped raise the standard of professionalism in the fitness industry and who have continually motivated me to strive for excellence in health and fitness education:

- Peter and Kathie Davis of IDEA, the International Association for Fitness Professionals
- Sheryl Marks Brown of ACE, the American Council on Exercise
- Peg Jordan, RN, and Linda Pfeffer, RN, of AFAA, the Aerobics and Fitness Association of America
- John McCarthy of IHRSA, the International Health, Racquet, and Sportsclub Association

Special thanks to all of our Brick Bodies "Semper Fi" staff, especially Erin Miller, for its dedication and commitment. I'd also like to acknowledge all of our Brick Bodies health club members, whose positive feedback, inspiration, and perspiration continually move me to help people improve the quality of their lives.

PART I

PREPARING FOR AEROBICS

Aerobic dance has changed a lot since the concept became popular in the late 1970s. At first, groups of people learned choreographed routines over six- to eight-week sessions. Classes were held at churches, recreation centers, racquet clubs, and schools. Today, aerobics has taken on a new meaning. Aerobics can be done in a group or by yourself, at home or in a health club. Aerobics routines today are not as choreographed. Routines have an organized flow, but they aren't performed so rigidly to the music. In addition, this exercise concept has broadened to include many different forms such as chair, low impact, hi/lo impact, interval, step, and slide aerobics. People have discovered that aerobics helps them feel and look better and obtain health benefits—all while they are having fun!

I have been involved in dance all my life, but after the birth of my first child I lost my stamina and my figure. My husband, who taught nutrition and aerobics classes to overweight women, approached me about teaching aerobics to his students. Although I had never taken an aerobics class before, I thought I could teach because I felt comfortable teaching dance choreography to people with various levels of experience. So my first aerobics class was the one that I taught.

Within two months I felt fantastic. My clothes fit, I felt more confident, and I had much more energy than ever before. And I still feel great, thanks to the regular aerobics fitness program I began some 14 years ago.

Today I own five health and fitness clubs. The clubs' mission is to provide a "magical experience" through quality service and fun fitness programs for all people, regardless of their ability or disability. Our members, guests, and I share a common goal: to improve our quality of life. But you don't have to be a member of a health club to gain the benefits of a regular aerobics program. All you need is a commitment to yourself.

Whether you are a seasoned aerobics enthusiast or a beginner, the workouts in *Fitness Aerobics* will help you to look and feel great. In part I, I will start you on your way with information that accomplishes these purposes:

- Explores the muscular strength, muscular endurance, and flexibility benefits you will notice within one month of beginning your regular aerobics program

- Discusses appropriate aerobics clothing, shoes, equipment, and music, and their respective estimated price tags, so you can get an appropriate start

- Helps you assess your readiness for aerobics, estimate your current fitness level, and determine the best level at which to begin

- Introduces you to the moves and terminology of the aerobics workouts in this book and helps you learn how to link movement combinations together so your aerobics workouts have an organized flow

- Describes appropriate warm-up and cool-down moves and stretches specific to each type of aerobics workout

Congratulations! You've taken the first step to improve the quality of your life. Enjoy the journey as you accomplish your goals.

1

Aerobics and Fitness

An aerobics program is one of the best ways for you to lose fat, increase muscle tone, and improve the quality of your life. Perhaps you are interested in starting your own program but you don't know where to begin. Maybe looking great and feeling good about yourself are your motivators. Or maybe you're already involved in a regular aerobics program and you're hungry for all the information you can get. This book is written to help all people to achieve their fitness goals, regardless of aerobics activity or location. In this chapter, I will address how to get started, how to add variety, and how to stick with your program. And best of all, you'll be able to begin your aerobics program today!

Why Do Aerobics?

We have learned a lot about exercise since the 1960s, when Dr. Kenneth Cooper defined aerobic fitness for the world. The fun but sophisticated aerobics classes that were so popular during the 1970s and 1980s have today been supplemented by a fitness industry that has standardized what is safe and unsafe and defined which workouts give the best results. This book offers a sampling of several very popular forms of aerobics: chair, low impact, hi/lo impact, step, interval, and slide. Aerobics workouts can be tailored to meet your individual tastes, specific fitness needs, and specific fitness goals.

The aerobics workouts in this book include aerobic "dance" as well as movement-oriented athletic conditioning. If you don't consider yourself to be a dancer, don't be intimidated. Aerobics exercise movements coordinate upper body and lower body together. They are much more fun and exciting for you when you combine basic movements that flow together.

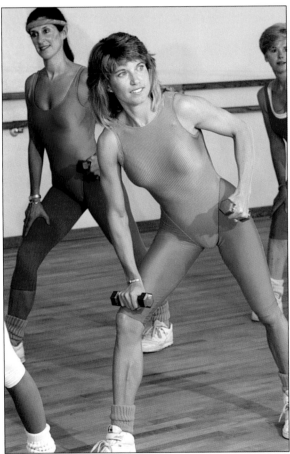

© F-Stock/David Stoecklein

The Physical Benefits of Aerobics

If you already do aerobics, then you know this kind of exercise makes you feel great. But what does it do for your body? Let's look at how aerobics benefits five aspects of physical fitness.

- **Cardiovascular.** The term *aerobic* means "with oxygen." Here's a quick physiology lesson: As you work out, your muscles need oxygen to work efficiently. As the muscle workload increases, your body responds by increasing the amount of oxygen it delivers to the muscles of the extremities and heart. Consequently, your heart rate and breathing rate increase to meet those demands. Oxygen is exchanged for carbon dioxide, which is then exhaled. Your body perspires, and you burn calories and fat.

  Aerobics improves your level of physical fitness and helps your body work more efficiently. The cardiopulmonary system (the heart, blood vessels, and lungs) is the primary system used by the body during an aerobic workout.

  Your body will adapt to your aerobics exercise program within a few weeks. You will find that your resting heart rate and blood pressure will lower, your heart will pump more blood with every beat, and you will develop more blood vessels to assist in delivering oxygen to the working muscles. The systems of the body work together to help improve your level of aerobic conditioning.

- **Muscular strength.** To become stronger, muscles must be worked beyond their normal loads. This is called the *overload principle.* To strengthen muscles, you must train at high intensity over a short time, using maximum resistance for a minimum number of repetitions.

  Don't expect significant strength gains from steady-state aerobics workouts where the intensity remains constant. You are more likely to gain strength during interval training, where the intensity level alternates from very high intensity to very low intensity exercise for several cycles. The low intensity exercise may incorporate forms of muscle endurance training with rubber bands, tubing, or light weights.

  Aerobics exercises that simulate strength training exercises (e.g., upright rows, triceps kickbacks, etc.) will help to shape and tone your muscles. If you incorporate a strength training program along with your aerobics program, your muscles will become stronger.

- **Muscular endurance.** Aerobic conditioning helps improve your muscular endurance. Muscular endurance is enhanced by performing maximum repetitions with minimum resistance. Aerobics activities, such as jumping jacks, knee lifts, and kicks, provide the repetitive movements needed to improve muscular endurance.

  The aerobics workouts in this book are designed to tone your muscles in the front of the body as well as the back, on the sides as well as the middle. Specific aerobics workouts focus on specific muscle groups. Chair aerobics primarily uses the upper body muscles; low impact, hi/lo, and interval aerobics use all muscles of the upper and lower body. Slide aerobics focuses on the inner and outer thigh as well as the hip flexor and quadriceps muscles. Step aerobics focuses on the hip flexor and quadriceps muscles because they are used to help you up to the top of the step. Because the muscles of the front of the leg are really worked, moves that utilize muscles of the back of the leg (hamstring curls, gluteal squeezes) must be incorporated within the step aerobics workout, so all the muscles of the body are strengthened. A well-balanced body reduces the risk of injury.

- **Flexibility.** *Flexibility* is the range of motion around a joint. After you finish your aerobics workout, stretching will help you improve your flexibility as well as help blood circulate back to your heart. Muscles are like rubber bands: The more you stretch them, the more elastic they become. When you consistently stretch after your workouts, you will find that your muscle and joint range of motion will increase.

- **Body composition.** The last component of physical fitness is *body composition*, which refers to the ratio of lean muscle mass, bone, and necessary fluids in your body compared to fat. A person who is thin and weighs little can still be overfat. On the other hand, a professional football player could weigh more than the standard height and weight charts recommend but still have only 4 percent body fat. Regular aerobics exercise will lead to changes in your body composition, reducing your body fat and toning your muscles.

  The most important thing to remember is that you cannot lose fat in only one area of your body. This fallacy is commonly referred to as spot reducing. Aerobics will help you reduce your overall body fat.

  Weight control is a concern for many people. The bottom line in understanding weight control is that energy intake (food) must be less than energy output (calories burned in your workout). Aerobic activities performed at low to moderate intensity for 30 minutes burn approximately 250 calories, or the number of calories in one soda. Aerobics performed at low to moderate intensity for 20 minutes or more will burn fat. High intensity aerobic activity performed in short durations (less than 20 minutes) will burn sugar.

Another Physical Benefit

Forms of aerobics, such as low impact, hi/lo, interval, step, and slide, provide many physical benefits. You can become physically "addicted" to aerobics fitness training. During aerobics, your body will naturally secrete hormones with pain-inhibiting qualities. This gives you the aerobics equivalent of a euphoric "runner's high." Your body becomes accustomed to this wonderful feeling, which in turn helps you maintain a consistent exercise program.

Comparing Aerobics to Other Fitness Activities

As you can see in the graph below, the benefits from aerobics compare favorably to other fitness activities. Almost every benefit is as strong if not stronger than the compared fitness activities. This is why aerobics is such a well-rounded fitness program.

Aerobics is one of the most popular forms of fitness training because it is so much fun and can be done alone or with other people. Aerobics workouts not only help you to feel better about yourself, they also help you sleep better, relieve stress, and allow you to have a great time while you are working out. What are we waiting for? Let's get moving!

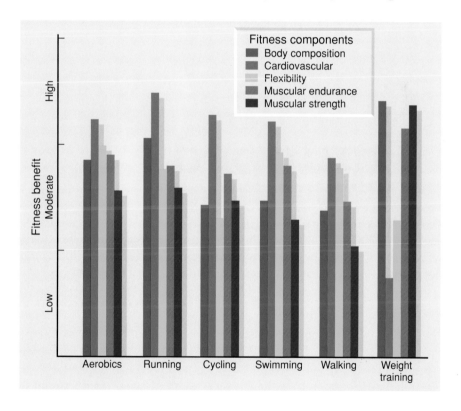

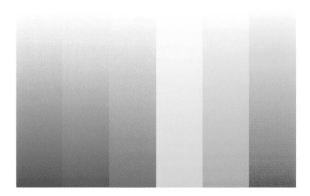

2

Getting Equipped

Aerobics is a great way to work out because it can be done spontaneously or with preparation. It is safe, effective, fun, and offers a lot of variety regardless of your experience level. It can be even more enjoyable if you take some time to prepare before you start. This chapter identifies what you should wear, what specific equipment you will need, environmental conditions for aerobics conditioning, and anticipated expenses.

Dressing Properly

How you choose to dress for aerobics is strictly personal and depends on your individual taste and budget. Almost anything goes, from a baggy T-shirt and gray sweat pants to a leotard with coordinating tights, sports bra, headband, belt, socks, and other accessories. The most important thing is that you feel comfortable while you are working out. Comfort starts with proper footwear.

Shoes

Your aerobics shoes need to be comfortable and provide support. Tennis or racquetball shoes may not offer a lot of cushion under the ball of the foot. Running shoes are not recommended because they are designed for forward movement only. Cross trainers may work, especially if you plan to wear them for other activities; however, they may feel heavy on your feet.

Aerobics shoes are designed specifically for aerobics exercise activities. All high impact aerobics require that you roll through the foot with a toe-ball-heel action. Therefore your shoes need to have good cushioning under the balls of your feet. Aerobics that require heel-ball-toe action, such as low impact aerobics, require shoes with heel support. Most aerobics programs today incorporate multiple impact activities (i.e., some low impact, some high impact, some step); therefore, shoes on the market today provide air cushioning, shock dispersion, heel pads, or energy return systems inside the shoe to give your toe, forefoot, and heel cushioning and support.

Aerobics requires a variety of movements. Kicks, jumps, jacks, marching, stepping, and twists are examples of different types of moves in which your feet land in different ways. Because your entire body weight is supported by your feet, shoes designed for aerobics offer a variety of supports to the outsides and the arches of the feet. Lateral support is provided by strips of leather, stitching, or fabric on the outside of the shoes.

The arch of the foot is supported with inserts made of foam, polyurethane, or other materials that are both supportive and resilient. These inserts can be removed for proper "airing out" after each use, which also helps to enhance the arch support's longevity. You need good arch support in aerobics shoes because every time you jump and land, the arch of your foot supports the weight of your entire body. (As a matter of fact, the force of your feet striking the ground is equal to about six times your body weight.) Without proper support, your arch will collapse, which can cause injuries to the muscles and/or joint structures surrounding the shin, knee, and hip.

Shoe manufacturers such as Avia, Reebok, Nike, Ryka, L.A. Gear, and Saucony make shoes specifically for aerobics that provide the proper amount of support and cushioning. One aerobics shoe product may differ from another in cut, design, and feel. To determine which shoe is best for you, you need to have a professional shoe representative or a podiatrist analyze your feet.

In the face of so many options, the best thing to do is to try on several pairs of aerobics shoes from a reputable shoe store and determine which pair feels best on your feet and provides the necessary support and cushioning. Different brands may feel different on your feet because of the shape of the foot and the cut of the shoe. What is best for you depends on your specific needs and your likes and dislikes. Many shoe stores may allow you to return shoes if you are not completely satisfied.

Comfort and support are the most important features when looking for good aerobics shoes. I recommend that you wear your aerobics shoes only

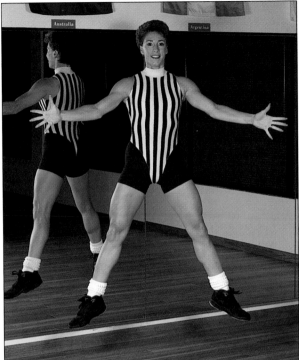

© Patrick Sandor/Sun Magazine

for aerobics to make them last. Most shoes last between three and six months if they are worn every day. Yes, you can wear them for gardening *after* they no longer give your feet support and cushioning when you do aerobics.

Clothes

Aerobics requires a lot of movement, so the clothes you choose to wear should be loose and allow you to feel comfortable as you sweat. Clothing that is very bulky is not recommended because it doesn't allow you or your instructor to monitor your body alignment. Leotards, tights, shorts, T-shirts, or lycra or spandex shorts are great for aerobics. Clothing and socks made of cotton will absorb perspiration and allow your skin to breathe as you work out.

Another very important item of clothing is proper athletic support. For protection, women should wear a bra designed for running, like the Jogbra, and men should wear appropriate athletic support that doesn't bind.

Dress in layers during cool weather. As you feel your body temperature rise, take off layers of clothing one at a time. For example, if the outside temperature is freezing or below, you may put on your leotard and tights, a T-shirt over that, then a full warm-up suit, then your outer layer of winter clothing. As your body temperature rises, take off your warm-up, then your T-shirt. After your workout, let your body temperature come down to normal (ideally you will take a shower and stop perspiring) and place the layers back on before you go back out into the cold weather.

Other Essentials

Once you have comfortable clothing and the proper footwear, consider a few more essential items:

- Water to replace fluids lost from aerobics. Water is the beverage of choice before, during, and after your workouts. Drink before you feel thirsty. Other beverages such as sodas, juices, or processed thirst quenchers will raise your blood sugar and affect the electrolyte balance in your body.
- Wristwatch to monitor your heart rate.

Optional Equipment

You might not need the following items if you are new to aerobics, but you may consider purchasing them as you become more involved. The last two items on the list are necessary if you plan to do the step or slide workouts in part II.

- A chair for chair aerobics. Arm rests are recommended if balance is a concern.
- A mat for cool-down stretching if you feel your carpeting does not provide enough cushioning. The mat should be approximately 36 inches by 48 inches and be made of foam or foam covered with cloth.
- A towel to wipe your perspiration.
- Rubberized tubing with handles, rubber bands, or one-, three-, and five-pound weights for interval aerobics.
- A step product or wood bench. Recommended dimensions are 6 to 8 inches high by 12 inches wide by 24 to 36 inches long.
- A slide board and slide booties or socks. The slide should be approximately four to six feet long and two to three feet wide. Slides are made of a slippery plastic material with angled rubber bumpers on either end. The booties or socks, made of a nonstick material, should fit over your shoes.

Environmental Conditions

Certain environmental conditions will enhance the safety of aerobics. The floor or surface that you work out on, air circulation, and the amount of space you need are factors that will make aerobics even more fun.

Suspended wood floors, carpeted and matted floors over wood (which can be found at most reputable health and fitness clubs), and grass surfaces are recommended for aerobics. Many manufacturing companies specialize in floor surfaces suitable for safe aerobics. These surfaces usually offer firm support while being resilient. Ideally, they have a base floor made of wood, then a solid piece of foam padding or foam blocks placed under sheets of wood, and a top layer of carpet or non-skid wood. If you have limited access to ideal floor surfaces, be sure to choose a different surface for each workout during the week. Thick wrestling or gymnastic mats (which have a lot of give but limited support) and concrete floors (which have a lot of support but no give at all) are not recommended.

You need at least 20 square feet of space to ensure that you have adequate room for full range of motion of your arms and legs. The ceiling of your fitness room should be 10 to 15 feet high—higher if you have ceiling fans—to allow enough clearance when you jump, even if you are using a step or bench product.

The temperature of your workout room should range between 65 and 72 degrees Fahrenheit—warm enough to allow you to perspire, yet cool enough to allow you to feel comfortable and not overheated. Many health

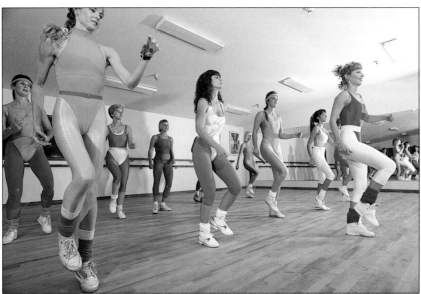

© F-Stock/David Stoecklein

clubs control the temperature with computer-controlled thermostats. In addition, the air should circulate to allow your perspiration to evaporate and help lower your body temperature. Ceiling fans, floor fans, and open windows help to circulate the air.

Music

Because aerobics is the coordination of music and movement, the music you choose should have the following features:

1. The beats per minute (BPM), which indicate the speed of the music, should be displayed. BPM are determined by counting the strongest beat over a one-minute period. The lower the BPM, the slower the music; the higher the BPM, the faster the music. The music's BPM should allow you to effectively work within your target heart rate range and allow you to get full range of motion. Recommended BPM safe ranges are given in the table below.

BPM Safe Ranges					
	Chair	**LIA and hi/lo**	**Interval**	**Step**	**Slide**
Warm-up	120-130	120-135	120-135	125-135	125-135
Aerobics	120-140	135-158	Alternate 3 minutes of 135-158 BPM with 1 minute of 120-126 BPM	118-126	120-126

2. The music should be fun, energizing, and have a driving beat. The music you choose to work out to will help inspire and motivate you. It can make your workout not seem like work!

3. Choose music that has 4 beats per measure and an even beat. Movements easily flow to the music when the music is written with 4 beats per measure and the phrasing of the music flows in 32-count increments. For example, 4 knee lifts (2 counts each) plus 8 marches or jogs equals 16 counts. Repeat this and you have 32 counts of movement that will flow with 32 counts of music.

A variety of music styles will help you choose a variety of movement styles. Music with a Latin theme will inspire you to do movements such as the cha-cha, mambo, or samba. Music of the sixties will inspire you to do movements reminiscent of the twist, the pony, and the jitterbug. Country music will get you in the mood for "The Achy Breaky" and other country dances. Music selections are suggested for each workout in part II. Audiocassettes of these selections can be obtained from the companies listed in appendix B.

Adding Up the Costs

An aerobics program can cost as little or as much as you feel is necessary. For example, time may be the only cost invested in a great aerobics workout in your home. On the other hand, if you choose to join a health club or fitness center, you can invest a large amount of money.

When you are designing your aerobics program it is wise to shop around for the best prices to suit your fitness goals. The following sample items are listed with their respective retail values.

Clothing	
Leotard	$20-30
Tights	$20-30
Bra top	$15-28
Belt	$6-10
Biker shorts	$15-20
Socks	$4-7
Headband	$3-5
Athletic support	$10-15

Shoes (price depends on the style and use)	
Aerobics	$60-115
Cross trainers	$50-120
Step	$60-105

Equipment	
Step	$30-130
Rubber tubing	$5-10
Rubber band	$3-6
Dumbbells (1-, 3-, 5-, 8-, 10-pound)	$10-100
Boogie box	$35-100
Slide board	$50-100
Audiocassette	$15-25
Mat	$15-25

Classes

Class fees vary depending on the type of program that is offered. Recreational programs, such as those offered by park districts, can cost as little as two or three dollars per class in an eight-week session. On the other hand, a health club membership that provides a variety of fitness classes plus other fitness programs and amenities can cost from 30 to 50 dollars per month. Some clubs offer a drop-in fee of 7 to 10 dollars per visit. Shop around for the type of aerobics program best suited to your needs. The staff should be certified by nationally recognized organizations such as the American College of Sports Medicine (ACSM), the American Council on Exercise (ACE), and the Aerobics and Fitness Association of America (AFAA). They should also be genuinely concerned about improving the quality of your life.

The amount of time you invest depends on your fitness goals and your current level of fitness. The time you dedicate to your aerobics program is as important as the time you dedicate to eating, sleeping, and other essential activities of daily living. Remember, "Those who think they have not time for bodily exercise will sooner or later have to find time for illness" (Edward Stanley).

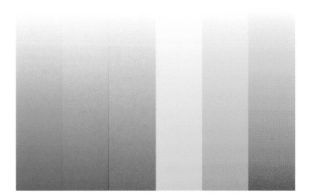

Checking Your Aerobic Fitness

Now that you're equipped for aerobics, you're probably wondering exactly how to begin. To determine which aerobics workout zones to choose from, whether you are a novice or advanced aerobics enthusiast, you'll first need to test your present level of health and fitness.

Health and *fitness* have two different meanings. Health refers to the absence of disease or injury. Fitness, on the other hand, is the ability to perform a specific physical task. You could be healthy but unable to meet the physical demands of aerobics. Or you may have the capability to perform an intense aerobics workout but be medically unhealthy.

I realize that most people really don't want to take the time to check their present level of health and fitness, so I've made the tests in this chapter simple, fun, and easy to do. If you are a beginner, the results will help you determine where you should begin, help you determine the results you want, and most important, help you get a safe and effective start into aerobics. If you are an experienced aerobics enthusiast, the results will help you appropriately choose from the menu of aerobics workouts in part II. Be aware that the health and fitness tests in this chapter are only general measures. If you have any concerns at all, obtain a physician's physical exam or stress test.

Assessing Your Physical Readiness

Aerobics can be strenuous physical activity. Be honest with yourself as you answer the questions on the Preparticipation Checklist below and perform your fitness test. Overestimating your capabilities or ignoring key health items could prevent your aerobics success.

PREPARTICIPATION CHECKLIST

Do you now have or have you had in the past any of the following conditions?

Yes	No	
___	___	1. History of heart problems, chest pain, or stroke
___	___	2. Increased blood pressure
___	___	3. Any chronic illness or condition
___	___	4. Difficulty with any physical exercise
___	___	5. Advice from a physician not to exercise
___	___	6. Surgery within the last 12 months
___	___	7. Pregnancy, now or within the last three months
___	___	8. History of breathing or lung problems
___	___	9. Any present muscle, joint, or back disorder, or any previous injury that still affects you
___	___	10. Diabetes or thyroid condition
___	___	11. Cigarette smoking habit
___	___	12. Obesity (more than 20 percent over ideal body weight)
___	___	13. Increased blood cholesterol
___	___	14. History of heart problems in your immediate family
___	___	15. Hernia, or any other condition that may be aggravated with physical activity
___	___	16. Any present condition that requires medications or drugs that can alter your ability to perform aerobics
___	___	17. Are you 40 years old or older (men)?
___	___	Are you 50 years old or older (women)?

Adapted, by permission, from The American Council on Exercise, 1991, *ACE Personal Trainer Manual* (San Diego: The American Council on Exercise), 141.

The Preparticipation Checklist gives a general indication of your state of health. Use it to determine if you have any health concerns that would contraindicate engaging in an aerobics program at this time. If you answer "yes" to any of the questions, consult your physician before you start aerobics or any other fitness program. If you answer "no" to all of the questions, it is generally safe to start your aerobics program.

Testing Your Aerobic Fitness

First, determine your activity level (0-7) by taking the Current Physical Activity Level test below. Record this number in the Personal Summary Box on page 22.

CURRENT PHYSICAL ACTIVITY LEVEL

Circle the number (0-7) that best describes your general activity level for the previous month.

I do not participate regularly in programmed recreational sport or heavy physical activity.

0   I avoid walking or exertion, such as by always using the elevator or driving whenever possible.

1   I walk for pleasure, routinely use stairs, and occasionally exercise sufficiently to cause heavy breathing or perspiration.

I participate regularly in recreation or work requiring modest physical activity such as golf, horseback riding, calisthenics, gymnastics, table tennis, bowling, weight lifting, or yard work.

2   I exercise from 10 to 60 minutes per week.

3   I exercise for more than one hour per week.

I participate regularly in heavy physical exercise such as running or jogging, swimming, cycling, rowing, skipping rope, running in place, or engaging in vigorous aerobic activity such as tennis, basketball, or handball.

4   I spend less than 30 minutes per week in physical activity, or run less than one mile per week.

---

5   I spend from 30 to 60 minutes per week in physical activity, or run from one to five miles per week.

6   I spend from one to three hours per week in physical activity, or run from 5 to 10 miles per week.

7   I spend more than three hours per week in physical activity, or run more than 10 miles per week.

Determining Your Heart Rate

To complete your fitness test, you need to know how to determine your heart rate. Your heart rate will also help you determine your exercise intensity during each aerobics workout.

Place your second and third fingers (never your thumb) along the thumb side of your wrist, between the bone and the tendon that you feel.

If you have difficulty finding your pulse at the wrist, you can feel your pulse along the side of your neck, between your voice box and the large neck muscle. Be sure to touch your neck gently as you count your pulse, because excessive pressure on the large artery in your neck can slow your heart momentarily.

Count every pulse you feel for 15 seconds. Multiply your count by 4 to find your one-minute heart rate. Measure your heart rate before you start your fitness test. The more you practice taking your heart rate, the easier it becomes.

Taking the STEP Fit Test

Step fitness testing procedures have been done by researchers at Harvard University since 1930 and have been regarded worldwide as a reliable test of fitness levels. The three-minute STEP Fit Test on page 20 will help you determine your aerobic fitness level. The STEP Fit Test is a standardized test that does not require you to work at high intensity levels.

Your STEP Fit Test score, combined with your Current Physical Activity Level score, will give you an estimate of your Relative Fitness Level. Locate

STEP FIT TEST

Equipment

1. An eight-inch high step, such as The STEP®, sturdy boards stacked together, or your steps at home.
2. A consistent quarter note beat (76 beats per minute) for three minutes. You can determine the beat in one of the following ways:

   - Use the second hand of your watch to assure that you complete five of the four-count sequences (up, up, down, down) in 15 seconds. You may want to practice before you take the test.
   - Set a metronome at a rate of 76 beats per minute and move your feet alternately every time the metronome clicks.
   - Use music that has a strong sense of pulse, beating 76 times per minute.

3. A watch with a sweep hand or a digital watch.

Directions

1. Enter a quiet room. The temperature should be between 65 and 75 degrees Fahrenheit. Rest for five minutes. Remove heavy clothing and wear comfortable shoes.
2. Warm up by marching in place for three to five minutes, then stretch. Pay special attention to stretching your calves, hip flexors, and hamstrings. See chapter 5 for specific stretches.
3. Start the tape or metronome that is set for 76 beats per minute.
4. Set your watch to begin counting three minutes.
5. Begin stepping up onto the step with an up, up, down, down routine. You can lead with the right foot up first, then switch to lead with the left foot. Be sure to place your entire foot up onto the step and roll through your foot with a toe-ball-heel action each time you step off.

   Stay on the beat of the music or in time with the metronome. If you cannot stay in time because of poor coordination or physical exhaustion, stop. Take the test again after several weeks.
6. When you complete three minutes of exercise, wait exactly 15 seconds, then take your pulse for exactly 15 seconds.
7. Take this heart rate and multiply it by 4 to obtain your one-minute heart rate. Record this number in the Personal Summary Box on page 22.

FITNESS STEPPING, © 1993, The STEP Company. Relative Fitness Levels are reproduced with permission. For a complete FITNESS STEPPING brochure with The STEP Fit Test and Fitness Stepping Prescriptions please send a self-addressed stamped envelope to The STEP Company, 2250 New Market Parkway, Suite 130, Marietta, GA 30067.

the Relative Fitness Level chart below for your age and sex, and record your score in the Personal Summary Box on page 22. These charts were designed for fitness stepping specifically, not for general fitness. Use them as guidelines only to give you an idea of your present level of aerobic fitness.

It does not matter whether you have a high, average, or low fitness level score. The results of your test are meant to help you determine which aerobics fitness program in chapter 13 is best for you.

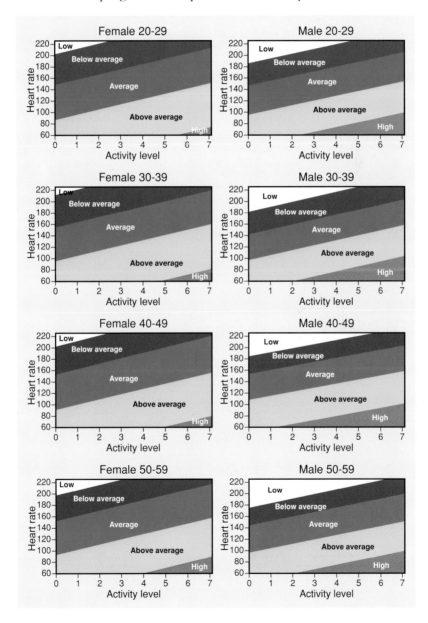

PERSONAL SUMMARY BOX

Current Physical Activity Level (0-7)　　　　_____

STEP Fit Test score (one-minute heart rate)　　_____

Relative Fitness Level (high . . . low)　　　　_____

One of the most common errors is miscalculating the heart rate. If you suspect a scoring error, retake the test another day. Also, you should not take this test

- after strenuous physical activity,
- immediately after you drink coffee or smoke,
- when you are anxious or excited, or
- in an extremely warm room (above 78 degrees Fahrenheit).

Feel free to retest yourself to reconfirm your fitness level or to see if your fitness level has improved through using the aerobics workouts that follow. The next chapter will help you do your fitness aerobics the right way.

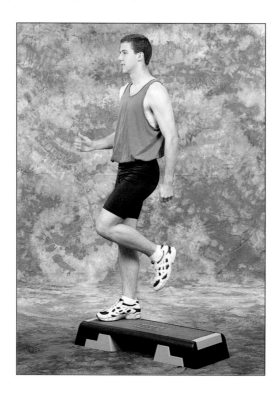

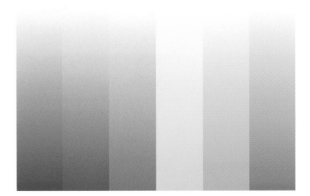

Aerobics the Right Way

Aerobics is a fun activity that is easy to do. However, just like all other forms of fitness training, the technique you use should help you get the most out of your workout without causing injury or stress to your body. In this chapter, we'll explore safe training techniques as well as the exercises and movements you should avoid.

You must first learn the components of correct posture and alignment. Although this may seem very basic, poor posture and alignment can be one of the major sources of injury or stress to the body from doing aerobics. Once your posture is in line, we'll look at other factors that can make or break a great fitness aerobics workout.

Fitness Aerobics Techniques

In the pages that follow, I provide specific descriptions of how to perform the movements used in the workouts in this book. A few general concepts apply to all of them, and I'll discuss those first.

Use Proper Posture and Alignment

Stand straight and tall with your head over your shoulders, your shoulders over your hips, your hips over your knees, and your knees over your feet.

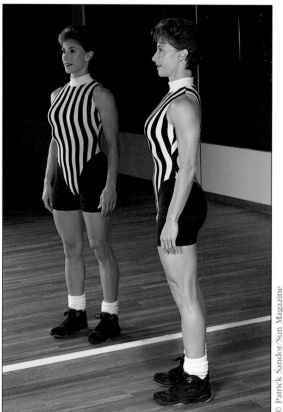

© Patrick Sandor/Sun Magazine

If you were to draw a plumb line along the side of your body, all of these bony parts should be in line.

Concentrate on keeping your stomach muscles tight, your shoulders back and relaxed, and your tailbone tucked in a neutral, or centered, position under your hips to help stabilize your back for all of your fitness activities. Practice lifting up from under your rib cage as you keep your chest open and your shoulders back and relaxed. Think of your chest as an open window. For men, your chest is your center of gravity, and the point from which balance and body control stem. For women, however, your center of gravity is located in your pelvic region because of your wider pelvic structure that allows you to bear children.

You may find that it's easiest to work on your posture and alignment if you exercise in front of a mirror so you can check your alignment from the front and side. After you've graduated from an aerobics fitness novice to an aerobics fitness enthusiast, you may not even need a mirror at all.

Keep your body aligned properly during every warm-up, exercise, and stretch. Practice good posture even when you are not working out, such as when you are driving, grocery shopping, or doing the dishes. The more you do this, the easier it will be for you to have great posture and alignment when you are exercising. Great posture and alignment help you project an image of self-confidence and success in all you do at work and at home. Soon, good posture and alignment will become second nature as you go about all of your daily activities.

Execute Moves Through the Full Range of Motion

Make each move have a beginning and an end. For example, a biceps curl starts with the hand alongside the body and ends with the hand at the shoulder. You will derive the most benefit if you work toward executing moves to their fullest and at the best of your ability.

Adjust the Impact

Many years ago, aerobics began as an exclusively high impact activity. The impact forces on the feet greatly stressed the ankles, shins, knees, and hips. Many participants were soon injured. As a result, low impact and moderate impact aerobics were born, along with chair aerobics, interval training, step training, and slide training. You'll find all of these types of aerobics fitness training activities in the workouts in this book. Combining low, moderate, and high impact movements in a workout is the safest and most effective technique for avoiding injury. Movement combinations vary the impact forces on the foot, ankle, knee, and hip.

Vary Movement Intensity

In general, low intensity moves are closest to the ground, moderate intensity moves are a little farther away from the ground, and high intensity moves are farthest away from the ground. This rule of intensity applies to the upper body as well as the lower body. For example, heel touches with biceps curls are low intensity upper and lower body moves. High kicks with the arms-overhead press are high intensity upper and lower body moves.

One way to increase intensity is to add one hop to a four-count movement. For example, hop on the fourth and eighth counts of a grapevine. In addition, if you make your movements travel, the intensity will increase. *Fitness Aerobics* workouts focus on providing specific intensity levels appropriate for the workout zone, but you can alter the intensity so the workout feels best for you.

Aerobics Moves

The descriptions and concepts of the following aerobics fitness moves are the basis for the workouts in part II, so take some time to learn them. Moves are listed alphabetically within the categories of chair, low impact aerobics (LIA), moderate impact aerobics (MIA), high impact aerobics (HIA), step, and slide. I describe arm movements that are used in all workout types (except slide) first. When moves can be done in either direction, I describe the movement to the right (R) only. Any move described this way (such as step touch R) can also be done to the left (L). Moves with a ◆ following their descriptions are illustrated in appendix A.

Arm Movements

Front raise. Both arms raise in the front of your body up to shoulder level on count 1 and lower on count 2.

Monkey. Alternate arms raise overhead then lower to the waist on every beat of the music.◆

Open and cross. Both arms lift to the side on count 1, then cross in front of the chest on count 2.◆

Pump. Both arms swing forward and back from the shoulder with the elbows slightly bent and at your sides, alternating on every musical beat. This is the same motion you generally use when you walk.◆

Punch. The fist punches either up, forward, across the body, or down. Can be done together (punch on count 1, return to start on count 2) or alternating (on every beat).

Sway. Both arms together swing side to side either low (at waist level) or high (above your head). On count 1 sway R, count 3 sway L.◆

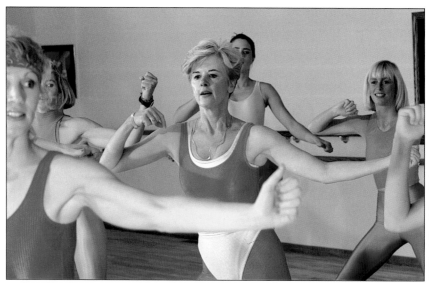

© F-Stock/David Stoecklein

Tap. Both hands tap on your thighs to make a slapping sound. Be careful not to hit yourself too hard!

Other arm movements will be used such as clap or hands on the thighs. You already know these moves.

Chair Aerobics

Chair aerobics is aerobics done while seated in a chair. The goal is to move as many muscle groups as possible to enhance aerobic benefits. Chair aerobics is most appropriate for people with balance or coordination concerns, pre- or postnatal women, maturing adults, a person with a low fitness level rating, or anyone who prefers to sit and be fit.

Any lower body movement that is done without traveling forward, back, or side to side can be easily transferred into a chair aerobics movement. Examples include the march, hop, step touch, touch step, knee lift, kick, and so on.

Upper body chair aerobics moves simulate the types of moves people do in a weight room with resistance apparatus. Moves can be done more slowly than the beat of the music (half time), on the beat of the music (single time), or faster than the beat of the music (double time). Both arms can move together or alternately. Upper body moves include the following:

Biceps curl. Start with your fists alongside your body with your palms facing forward. Bending your elbows, lift your fists up to your shoulders on count 1 and return to start on count 2.◆

Circles. Move either the fists or the forearms in *small circles*, or move the entire arm in *big circles*. Circles can be done low at side with fists or forearms alongside your body.

Lateral deltoid raise. With elbows bent and the upper arm alongside the body, lift your elbows laterally to shoulder height to do the *short lever* version of this move. The entire arm lifts out to the side up to shoulder height in the *long lever* version. Lift on count 1 and return to start on count 2.◆

Press. Lift one or both arms to shoulder level in front and press forward as if you're pushing something off your chest (also called *chest press*). The move can be done in single or double time. Variations include the *overhead press* (upward motion); *press down*◆ (downward motion); and *lateral triceps press* ◆ (lift elbow up to shoulder level with arm bent; hold elbow stationary while pressing forearm to the side).

Pull. Start with both arms straight down in front. Pull up so the elbows are bent and the fists are at the chin on count 1, then return to the straight lowered position on count 2. This is called an *upright row* ◆. Variations include the *pull down* ◆ or *lat pull down,* (starting with your arms over-head, pull the elbows down behind your back); *pull back high* (starting with elbows extended at shoulder level, pull in so your fists are at your chin), *pull back low* ◆ (start with arms extended at waist level; pull in toward waist). The arms can move together or one at a time.

Triceps kickback. Start with your elbows lifted and toward the back wall. Extend your forearm toward the back wall on count 1, then return to the original position on count 2.◆

Low Impact Aerobics

Low impact aerobics (LIA) movements require that you keep one foot on the floor at all times. Research proves that you burn just as many calories during LIA as you do during high impact aerobics (HIA) without the high level of stress to your joints. Here are examples and descriptions of low impact moves:

Cha-cha-cha. Step on your right foot, step quickly on the ball of your left foot, then step on your right foot again. The rhythm is step (count 1), ball (count &), change (count 2).

Grapevine R. Step your R foot to the R, cross the L foot back, step the R foot R, tap the L toe alongside of the R foot. *Grapevine L* is the reverse.

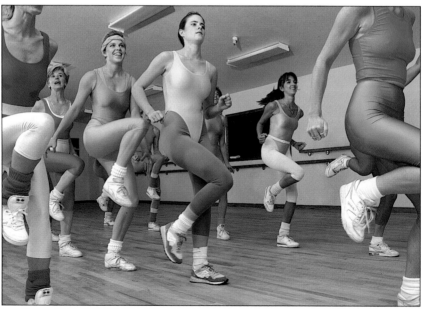

Knee lift. Do a 2-count movement in which the knee lifts on count 1 and the foot lands on the floor on count 2.◆ Variations include the *kick forward* from the knee, *kick rear* from the hip, and *hamstring curls.*◆

Lunge. Your hips turn to face the L wall as your R toe taps to the R wall on count 1. Your feet and hips come together on count 2 and reverse with the left foot.◆

Mambo. The R foot steps forward (count 1), the L foot steps on the spot (count 2), the R foot steps back (count 3), the L foot steps on the spot (count 4).

March. Lift your knees high as you walk, with each foot stepping on each beat of the music. One foot remains in contact with the floor at all times. As you bring each foot back to the floor, roll through your foot with a toe-ball-heel action.

Shuffle. For this succession of ball-changes, step on the R foot (count 1), the ball of the L foot (count &), R foot (count 2), the ball of the L foot (count &), R foot (count 3), the ball of the L foot (count &), R foot (count 4), and kick the L foot forward (count &). Continue the sequence by leading with the L foot.

Slide-slide-ball-change R. Step to the R with your R foot on count 1. Slide your L foot in to meet your R foot on the & count. Step your R foot to the R on count 2. Step back with the ball of the L foot (count 3), step the R foot on the spot (count 4). Reverse the sequence to the L.

Squat. Start with your feet flat on the floor and under your hips, then bend your knees. Can also be done to the right or left.◆

Step touch R. Step with your R foot to the right, then tap your L foot alongside your R foot. Reverse the movement with *step touch L.* Can also be done to the front or back.

Touch step R. Touch your R toe or heel to the side, front, or rear, then bring it back to center, placing your weight on your R foot as you place it next to your L foot. You can also do the movement with the L toe or heel (*step touch L*).◆

Triplet. In this rhythmic variation of step touch, step to your R with your R foot (count 1) then tap the ball of your L foot alongside of your R foot, keeping your body weight centered as you transfer your weight onto the ball of your L foot (count &). Transfer your weight onto your R foot (count 2). Reverse the sequence as you step with your L foot.

V step. Step your R foot forward diagonally R and then your L foot forward diagonally L. Step back at the same angle with your R foot and then step back at the same angle with your L foot.◆

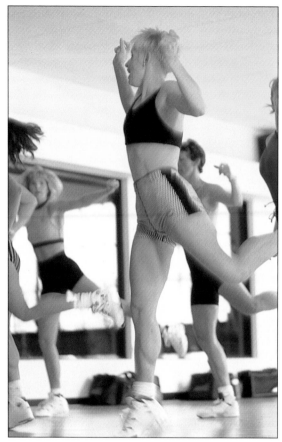

Courtesy of AVIA

Moderate Impact Aerobics

Moderate impact aerobics (MIA) moves refer to moves where the heel lifts, but the toes do not leave the floor. You feel as if you are jumping, but you're not. The following are examples of moderate impact moves:

Press up. Start with your feet under your hips, then raise up onto your toes. Bend your knees slightly as you lower your heels back to the floor.◆

Skip. Roll through the bottom of your feet with a toe-ball-heel action.◆

Twist. Keep your toes on the ground under your hips, lift your heels off the ground, and move your hips from side to side.

Any move that can be executed between low and high impact. For example, knee lifts can be done with the feet flat (low impact) or with the supportive foot hopping off the ground (high impact). In the moderate impact version of the same move, only the heel would lift up and down.

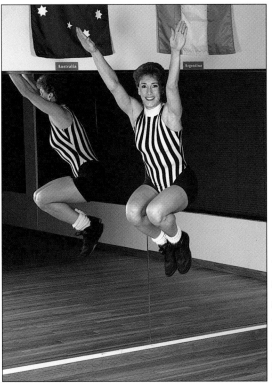

© Patrick Sandor/Sun Magazine

High Impact Aerobics

High impact aerobics (HIA) refers to moves in which the feet leave the floor. Impact forces on the feet are three to four times the body weight when the feet return to the floor. This force could eventually cause injury to the feet, ankles, shins, knees, and hips. But, when high impact moves are executed with proper techniques and are combined with low and moderate impact moves, they are safe, fun, and easy to do. Examples of high impact moves include the following:

Hop. One or both feet lift only one-half to two inches off of the floor.

Jack. Jump up, pushing both feet out, and land on count 1, then jump again, bringing both feet back together to land on count 2.◆

Jog. This is the landing technique for any high impact move. Lift your right foot off of the floor as you lift your right knee in front of your body. As you bring your right foot back to the floor, roll through your foot with a toe-ball-heel action every time. If the heel doesn't touch the floor every time, the calf will remain contracted and the Achilles tendon will remain shortened, which can cause stress to the heel, ankle, and shin. Repeat the same process with the left foot.

Jump. Both feet leave the floor and both feet land together.◆

Knee lift. The R knee lifts on count 1 as the supportive foot (L) leaves the floor. The R foot lands on count 2, then the sequence continues with the L knee.◆ Any variation of a leg lift, such as the kick, hamstring curl, or kick rear, is done with the same counts.

Lunge hop. This is a high impact variation of step touch. Step R foot forward (count 1) and jump up. As you land (count 2), bring your feet together, and either tap your L foot or place your L foot flat on the floor with your body weight evenly distributed. Continue this sequence with the L foot.◆

Power moves. Power moves are for advanced high impact exercisers. They take the entire body up off of the ground as high as you can jump. They also cause the hip to flex or bend as the knee lifts up toward your chest. They are great advanced options, especially for interval training. However, they must always accompany low impact moves to reduce the risk of injuries. Examples include the *power step touch, power heel tap front, power touch step*, and *power jump*. The *power slide, power jog*, and *power jack* each require one complete repetition for 4 musical counts.

Slide. Step your R foot to the side (count 1), jump up and bring your L foot in to meet your R foot (count &), then step your R foot out the side again after landing on your L foot (count 2).

Split. Jump up and land with one foot forward and the other foot back. Then jump and switch feet.◆

Twist. A move similar to the moderate impact twist. The feet can leave the floor but the feet should land under your hips to protect your back.

Step Aerobics

Step aerobics is a low impact, varied intensity activity that involves stepping up onto and off of a step product, bench, or stool. Here are a few step training tips:

- Use good posture and alignment. As you step up, lean with your entire body from the heel toward your head. Your tendency will be to lean forward from your waist as you step up.

- Step with your whole foot onto your step. Never let your heels hang off. Keep your knees slightly bent and aligned over your toes as you raise up onto your step.

- Step off with a toe-ball-heel action, allowing your heels to touch the ground each and every time. Never jump off! Place your feet between six and eight inches away from your step as you step off.

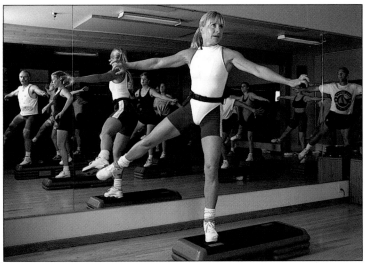

© F-Stock/Kirk Anderson

- Have one foot lead for a maximum of one minute. The lead foot is the foot that first steps onto or off of your step.

- When you're leading from the top (standing up on your step then stepping down), step down and back as you step off. Then step forward as you step back on top. Lunges and squats leading from the top should also be executed this way, stepping back first. This prevents stress and potential injury to the knee.

- Go slowly, especially if you're new to step training. It may initially feel difficult and awkward, but it becomes easier the more you do it.

The **basic lead (L or R)** is the primary move of step aerobics. To perform the basic R lead, step up onto your step with your R foot, step up with your L foot, step back down with your R foot, then step back down with your L foot. You may also lead with your L foot. It's as easy as that! The basic step can be done from any positioning to the step (for example, the middle or the end) whether the lead is from the floor or the top.

Following are the other step training moves you'll find in the workouts:

A step. Standing next to your step facing the L wall, step up with your R foot toward the end of the step, then step up with your L foot. Step down and back with your R foot, then down with your L foot on the opposite side of your step.◆

Across the top. This is a grapevine over the length of the step. Start at the L lateral side of your step. Step R foot up in center of step, L foot up together, step R foot down R lateral side of step, tap L foot down. Reverse by leading with the L foot.◆

Corner to corner. Starting from the corner at the end of your step, step up with your R foot to the center of the step, bring your L foot up together. Step down with your R foot off the opposite corner.◆

L step. Start at the far L side of your step behind your step. Step R foot up, tap L toe up, step L foot down along the L side, tap R foot down next to L foot. R foot up, L toe taps up, L foot steps down, R foot steps down (travel to R side of step). Now lead with the L foot. This move can be done with 3 knee lifts or with a combination of 1 knee lift, 1 heel tap up, 1 knee lift instead of tap up or down.◆

Lunge. Starting on top of the step, touch R foot on the floor behind the hips (count 1), touch together on top (count 2), touch L foot on the floor (count 3), feet together on top (count 4).◆

Over the top. This is a grapevine over the narrow side of the step. Face the L wall. Step up on your step with your R foot, step your L foot up together. Step down with your R foot on the opposite side, tap your L foot down on the floor. Continue by leading with the L foot.◆

Power moves. These advanced step moves make your body lift high off the ground by forcing the legs to push hard off the floor. They include the *power tap up, power knee lift, power abductor leap, power V step,* and *basic run step.*

Squat. Leading from the top, step down off with R foot (counts 1 and 2), step back up (counts 3 and 4). Reverse L lead (counts 5 through 8). Leading from the floor, squat up (2 counts), put feet together (2 counts), squat down (2 counts), tap down. Can also be done up, leading from the floor.◆

Straddle. This sequence involves the basic step leading from the top or the floor, with the step in between your legs.

T step. Begin this 8-count movement from the end of your step. From the floor, the R foot steps up, L foot steps up, R foot steps straddle down astride, L foot steps straddle down astride. R foot steps up, L foot steps up, R foot steps down back, L foot steps down back.◆

Tap down. With your R foot leading from the top of your step, step down with your R foot, tap your L toe down, and step up. Then with your L foot, tap your toe up. Repeat or alternate.

Tap up. This is the opposite of the tap down sequence. Step up with R foot, tap the L foot up onto the step. Then step down with your L foot, tap your R foot down. Repeat or alternate lead feet. This is the basic move for lower body variations. Instead of tapping your toe on top of the step, lift the leg forward, side, or rear. Examples include the *knee lift* ◆, *gluteal squeeze* ◆ (the entire leg lifts behind), *abductor lift* ◆ (leg lifts laterally), *hamstring curl* ◆ (the heel lifts up toward the buttocks), and *kick* (the leg kicks usually no higher than knee level).

Turn step. A variation of an alternate-foot tap down where you turn your shoulders and hips. As you step up with your R and L foot, turn your hips and shoulder to face the R wall. Reverse with the L foot leading.◆

V step. This is a wide basic step. Step R foot up wide, step L foot up wide, step R foot down to starting spot, step L foot down.◆

Slide Training

Slide training is high intensity lateral training that resembles sliding across your newly waxed kitchen floor in your stockinged feet. It utilizes a slide board that has angled, rubberized bumpers on either end of a slippery plastic material. Slide booties or socks are worn over your supportive shoes. The bumpers are angled for two reasons. The first is to help protect your knees. If your body were to slide into a straight bumper, your ankle, knee, and hip would try to cushion the impact. The angled deceleration ramp helps you slow your movement down and provides protection to your ankle, knee, and hip. The second reason is so you can push off of that bumper. It is much easier to push your foot off of a bumper that's angled than to push off of something that's flat. Your foot must be on top of the bumper before you attempt to push off, however.

Slide training is an advanced aerobics activity that requires skill, awareness of your body's position in space, balance, coordination, and physical readiness. It's often used for sport-specific training such as skiing, tennis, in-line skating, and speed skating. Slide training requires twice the energy expenditure of walking and helps develop the muscles of the lower body that are not often used with other forms of aerobic fitness. Slide training also helps improve balance and coordination. Remember these slide training tips:

- Place your slide board on a flat surface. The bumpers should be angled so that the top corners are farther away from the center of the board than the bottom corners are.

- Use good posture and alignment. Keep your knees over your toes and your eyes focused forward. Slide training requires a ready stance, which is the typical stance used for most sports.

- As you approach the bumpers, try to let the bottoms of your feet lift slightly outward toward the side wall. This will help you to place your feet up onto the bumpers.

- Secure your foot on top of the bumper whenever you do movement variations such as knee lifts, squats, or lunges.

The **basic slide** is an 8-count movement in which you slide 4 counts R, 4 counts L. Starting with the feet open, close them together, open them, then close them together again as you slide R then L. The basic slide R lead starts at the L side with the L foot placed on top of the bumper. Bend your

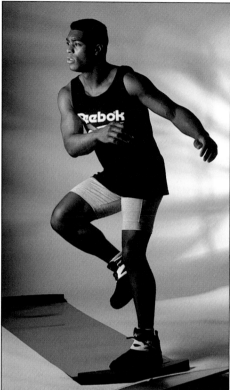

Courtesy of Step Reebok

knees and push off of the L bumper with your L foot (drag foot). Try to slide all the way to your R bumper with one push. If you cannot get there in one push, keep practicing this basic move until you can. Be sure to open your feet in the middle of the slide and close your feet at the bumpers. Now check your R foot placement. It should be on top of your bumper. Then reverse the movement, traveling back to your L bumper. The R basic slide and the L basic slide together comprise one slide stroke.

The following are other slide moves you'll find in the workouts:

Adductor slide. In the center of your slide, slide both feet out laterally at the same time; then slide back in together. This may feel more comfortable if you rotate your hips outward as you slide out, then squeeze in through your inner thighs and turn your feet parallel as you slide back together. The adductor slide can be done in four speeds: very slow (4 counts out, 4 in), slow (2 counts out, 2 in), fast (1 count out, 1 in), or double time (1 count for out and in).◆

Athletic (low profile) slide. Similar to the basic slide, the hips stay low in this movement, which is usually done in 2 counts R and 2 counts L. However, the feet do not close; rather, they remain in a wide stance.◆

Corner to corner. This sequence is similar to the step training move with the same name. Start at the back L side of your slide with your L foot placed on the L bumper. Push in a "telemark" fashion toward the R front corner. Secure your R foot at the R bumper.◆

Cross country. Similar to HIA splits. One leg pushes forward as the other leg pushes back. This can be done slowly (2 counts) or fast (1 count). Cross country can be done against the bumper, in the center of your slide, or even traveling.◆

Diagonal lunge. Stand in the center of your slide. Angle R foot toward the R front corner and slide your L foot back in 2 counts. Then slide the feet together in 2 counts.◆

Lunge. This movement can be done laterally to the side or to the rear facing the bumper. Be sure to keep your knee over your ankle.◆

Slide squat. This is the basic slide with the R foot leading in 2 counts, then squat 2 counts. Continue by leading with the L foot.◆

Stationary skating slide. Starting in the center of your slide, push and extend your R foot against the slide surface as it moves laterally. Then return to the starting position. Continue the movement with your L foot.◆

Tap. The toe taps on the floor. The tap can be done in front of or behind the slide board.◆

Telemark. This sequence starts at the L bumper, facing the R wall. The R foot is placed forward toward the middle of the board. Push your L foot on the L bumper and slide the R foot straight to the R bumper. The R foot remains forward and the L foot remains back. To reverse, turn your body to face the L wall and push off the R bumper.◆

Interval Training

Interval training alternates intervals of high intensity hi/lo aerobics with muscle conditioning. Usually, three to four minutes of high intensity aerobics training, which may also include power aerobics moves, are alternated with one to two minutes of active recovery, which is the muscle conditioning segment. Try to push yourself physically as hard as you can during your high intensity peaks so that when you recover, you'll feel as if you're resting.

You won't be resting too easily, however. Instead, you'll be in *active recovery*, where the lower body continues to circulate blood by doing some type of movement, such as squats, lunges, leg lifts, or marches. Meanwhile, the upper body may be doing some type of conditioning with or without weights, rubber bands, rubber tubing, or your other hand for resistance. Continue repeating the muscle conditioning activity for the allotted time during the workouts in the Orange and Red zones.

Interval training is a great way to burn calories and fat because you're tricking your body into a higher level of intensity without consistently maintaining an intensity level that could potentially cause injury.

Learning the Moves

The *link method* is the part-to-whole method of learning a skill or movement that makes learning complex skills much easier. By breaking the movement down into smaller, simpler parts, it is much easier to coordinate the upper body with the lower body. Each move is added gradually, one step at a time. For example, consider the following step combination:

Counts	Lower body	Upper body
1-8	Basic R lead × 2	Pull back low × 4
9-16	V step R lead × 2	Lateral deltoid raise × 4
17-24	Basic L lead × 2	Pull back low × 4
25-32	V step L lead × 2	Lateral deltoid raise × 4
33-128	Repeat × 3 more sets	

Start the combination by doing the lower body basic R lead. When you feel comfortable with that movement, add your upper body pull back low. Repeat the basic R lead with the pull back low until you feel absolutely comfortable.

Repeat this process for the next combination. Do the V step R lead until you've mastered it, then add the upper body lateral deltoid raise. Then combine the basic step with the V step, and accompany both moves with the appropriate arms. You may want to do four repetitions of each basic move, then only two as the combination indicates. Repeat this process for each lower body and upper body component.

Once you have completed all the movements, broken the movements into the designated counts, added the upper body movements if they feel comfortable, and you feel you have mastered the combination, then repeat the entire combination two to four times as the choreography indicates. Repeat the entire process with the second combination using the part-to-whole method.

Repeat the whole combination 1 (basic R lead and pull back low) and the whole combination 2 (V step R lead and lateral deltoid raise). Repeat the part-to-whole process for combination 3. Go back and repeat the whole combination 1, 2, and 3. Continue to do so for all combinations in each workout.

After you have learned and repeated each combination, you should then try to smoothly flow from one combination to the next. The choreography is specifically designed to help you do this. Repeat each series of linked combinations over and over within each zone for the designated amount of time. You'll reap the benefits of aerobics as you flow through the combinations.

Have Fun!

Aerobics fitness requires some skill, but the most important component to your workout is fun! Your workout should be so enjoyable that you'll want to do it again. Think of your workout as being a "fun-out," not a workout. You should do what *you* like to do. There are so many options waiting for you to explore.

To get the most benefit from your aerobics workout, remember to do it right and have a great time. Now you're ready for warming up and cooling down techniques for specific types of aerobics workouts.

5

Warming Up and Cooling Down

Your warm-up and cool-down are just as important as the workout itself. In this chapter you'll find the latest warm-up and cool-down techniques to perform before and after your aerobics workouts. Be sure to include a good warm-up and cool-down with every workout. These warm-up and cool-down techniques will help you get the most out of every aerobics workout.

Five Reasons to Warm Up

The warm-up is your physical, psychological, and emotional preparation for the workout.

Here are five reasons to warm up:

1. **Warm-up gradually elevates your heart rate.** The rhythmic movements performed during the warm-up start small and gradually become larger to elevate the heart rate. They are similar to the aerobics movements of your workout.

2. **Warm-up prepares your muscles and joints.** It's helpful to divide the upper and lower body into these planes of space: anterior (front), posterior (back), and mediolateral (middle and side). Movements addressing each of these planes of space will adequately warm up every major muscle group and joint so that none are accidentally omitted.

3. **Warm-up increases your core body temperature.** At the end of your warm-up, your body should feel warm and you should be sweating lightly. This state of readiness can be reached within six to eight minutes.

4. **Warm-up increases your fluid circulation.** As your movements gradually increase in intensity, so will the amount of blood that circulates to the working muscles and keeps your joints well lubricated.

5. **Warm-up prepares you psychologically and emotionally.** No one is always in the mood to work out, but you can begin every workout with a positive mental attitude (PMA). Start every workout by telling yourself how great you will feel when you're finished. Remind yourself of all the benefits you will obtain by taking this time for yourself. At the end of your workout you should feel proud of yourself for taking another step toward your aerobics goal. Before you know it, this PMA will carry over into your life at work and at home.

Warm-Up Sequencing

Your warm-up movements should be specific to the aerobics activities you'll be performing during your workout. It is not necessary to spend a lot of time warming up. The following sequence of movements is a great warm-up for aerobic activities:

1. **Center your body.** See "Use Proper Posture and Alignment" on page 23.

2. **Take two to four deep breaths.** These are also called *cleansing breaths* because they encourage deep exchange of oxygen and carbon dioxide in the lungs. Cleansing breaths help you relax and mentally prepare for your workout.

3. **Do four to eight back releases.** Bend your knees slightly and place your hands on your thighs to support your back as shown on page 42. Tuck your tailbone under and hold the position for one to two seconds. Move your tailbone back to the center, then let your tailbone stick out behind you. Move back to center. Repeat this a few more times.

4. **Now, move!** Turn on your favorite music and start by bending your knees to the rhythm. Add upper body moves such as the biceps curl. Change your feet to a march. Then change your upper body move to the chest press. You can do any variety of moves that you like. Choose movements that incorporate all planes of space so that you prepare every major muscle group and joint. Mix and match the upper body and lower body moves as suggested in each specific warm-up to give yourself a lot of variety and style.

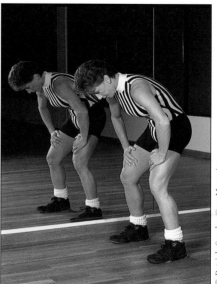
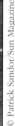
© Patrick Sandor/Sun Magazine

5. **Perform static stretches.** Hold static stretches in the warm-up for only 10 to 15 seconds. If you hold the stretches for long periods of time during the warm-up (as you will during the cooldown phase), the benefits of warming up that you worked so hard to obtain will be lost. Keep the upper body moving as you stretch the lower body without bouncing to ensure that your heart rate remains elevated. The major muscles to stretch during the warm-up are the calf, hip flexor, quadriceps, and hamstring muscles.

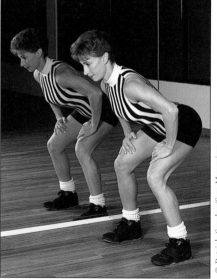
© Patrick Sandor/Sun Magazine

6. **Do toe taps.** Toe taps help strengthen the muscles, tendons, and ligaments that support the ankle and shin, to prevent shin splints. The muscles of the shin are usually much smaller than the calf muscles, and this muscle imbalance is what causes shin splints.

Warming Up for Specific Workouts

Follow the suggested warm-up moves that are appropriate for the specific workouts in part II. Perform 8 to 32 repetitions of each of the suggested moves. When you have completed the warm-up, your body should feel ready to work out.

Chair Warm-Up

Begin by sitting forward and tall in your chair and taking three to four deep breaths, then do low intensity upper body moves such as the biceps curl, press down, and press forward. Gradually increase intensity with lateral deltoid raise, small circles, and pull back high. Then do the pull down or overhead press. Next perform lower body moves such as the march, kick, or hop (you're still seated) while doing the upper body moves. Continue for approximately 4-1/2 minutes. Use music with 120 to 130 beats per minute (BPM). Finally, do upper back and front shoulder stretches.

Hi/Lo Warm-Up (Appropriate for LIA, Hi/Lo, and Interval Training Workouts)

Stand straight and tall as described in chapter 4. Begin by taking two to four deep breaths, then do four to eight back releases. Now march, step touch, touch step, and squat. Add upper body moves such as the biceps curl, press forward, press down, and lateral deltoid raise. Then alternately lift your knees and do the V step and grapevine with big circles, overhead press, and pull down. Continue for approximately 4-1/2 minutes with music at 120 to 135 BPM.

   Stretch your calf, hip flexor, quadriceps, and hamstring muscles.

Step Warm-Up

Begin by standing behind your step and taking two to four deep breaths, then do four to eight back releases. Now march, step touch, touch step, and squat. Add upper body moves such as the biceps curl, press forward, press down, and lateral deltoid raise. Then alternately lift your knees and do the V step and grapevine with big circles, overhead press, and pull down. Next do hamstring curls. Alternately tap your toe on top of the step, march on the step, and march off of the step so that you become aware of the step height and boundaries. Continue for approximately 4-1/2 minutes with music at 125 to 135 BPM.

   Stretch your calf, hip flexor, quadriceps, and hamstring muscles.

Slide Warm-Up

Stand behind your slide with the posture described in chapter 4. Begin by taking two to four deep breaths, then do four to eight back releases. Now march, touch step, and squat. Add upper body moves such as the biceps curl, press forward, press down, and lateral deltoid raise. Next do step touch slowly in order to simulate the basic slide motion. Then alternately lift your knees and do the grapevine with big circles, alternate press, and pull down. Continue for 4-1/2 minutes with music at 125 to 135 BPM.

Stretch your calf, hip flexor, quadriceps, and hamstring muscles. Put on your slide socks or booties. Continue to warm up as you begin basic slide training. Gradually increase intensity and continually check foot placement.

Cooling Down

After you have finished your aerobics workout, it is important to help your body return to its preworkout state. The best way to do this is by doing the same activities that you did to raise your heart rate.

In the first part of your cool-down, you will gradually decrease the movement intensity by doing 8 to 32 repetitions of simple moves on the spot (OTS). Your heart rate will gradually return to where it was before your workout began. Continue to use aerobics music for the first part of the cool-down.

The second part of cooling down involves stretching. The most important time to stretch all of your muscles is immediately following your workout, especially the ones that you specifically worked. For example, a step cool-down incorporates hip flexor and quadriceps stretches because the hip flexors are used every time you step up onto your step. You should also stretch the calf and hamstring muscles.

Stretching helps the blood circulate back to your heart, helps decrease your risk of injury, and helps you relax. You can continue to use aerobics music for stretching, or you can use any piece of music that is slow (less than 118 BPM) and relaxing.

Cooling Down for Specific Workouts

Following is suggested cool-down sequencing for the workouts in part II.

Chair Cool-Down

Decrease your movement intensity by doing the lateral deltoid raise, biceps curl, and press down. Slow each movement so you are performing each repetition in twice the amount of time.

Next, stretch your upper body with upper back, triceps and shoulder, front of shoulder, and chest stretches.

Hi/Lo Cool-Down (Appropriate for LIA, Hi/Lo, and Interval Workouts)

Gradually decrease your movement intensity by performing the march, step touch, touch step, and slow squats OTS.

Next, complete each of the nine lower body and upper body stretches.

Step Cool-Down

Gradually decrease your movement intensity by doing the basic right lead, basic left lead, tap up, and march on the floor.

Next, stretch your lower body, especially your hip flexor and quadriceps muscles as well as the lateral thighs and spine. Be sure also to stretch your upper body muscles. You can use the step as you stretch to hold onto or place your foot on, as you would when doing the vertical hamstring stretch.

Slide Cool-Down

Gradually decrease your movement intensity by slowing the basic slide then eventually holding a stationary position.

Next, remove your socks or booties and perform all of the lower and upper body stretches, focusing on the calf, hip flexor and quadriceps, and inner thigh muscles.

The nine stretches that follow will help make your warm-up and cool-down complete.

Calves

Stand with your feet shoulder width apart. Keep your toes and hips facing the same direction as you place one foot behind your hips. Gently lean forward so that you are straight from your head to your heel. Repeat with the other leg.

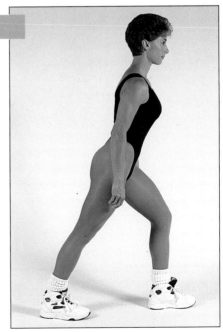

© Patrick Sandor/Sun Magazine

Hip Flexors and Quadriceps

Stand straight with your left foot on the floor. Place the shoelaces of your right foot into the palm of your right hand. Raise your left arm overhead or hold onto a chair for balance. Press your right knee toward the ground as you tuck your hips under. You should feel this stretch from your knee up to your hip. Repeat with your left leg.

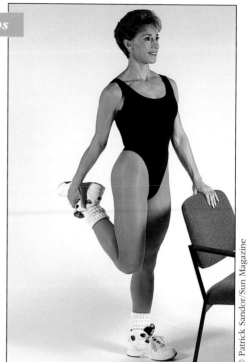

© Patrick Sandor/Sun Magazine

Inner Thighs

Using a wide stance and keeping your right knee over your right ankle, lean toward the right. Your right knee should be bent at greater than a 90-degree angle, your left leg should be straight, and your toes should face forward. You should feel this stretch in the left inner thigh. Now sit back into your right hip, supporting your back by placing your hands on your right thigh. Repeat on the left side.

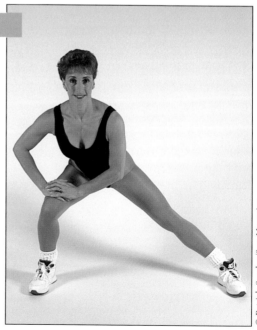

© Patrick Sandor/Sun Magazine

Hamstrings

Place your right heel into the ground. Step back with your left foot, keeping your feet shoulder width apart. Lift your chest and tilt your tailbone up as you lengthen your spine. Let your weight transfer to your left foot so that you feel the back of your right leg lengthen. Be sure to keep your right knee relaxed as you are stretching your hamstring muscles. Keep your hands on your thighs to support your back. Repeat with your left leg.

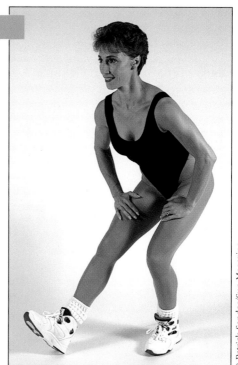

© Patrick Sandor/Sun Magazine

Lateral Thighs and Back

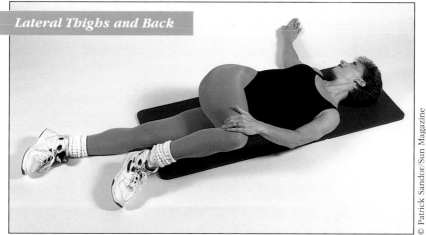

© Patrick Sandor/Sun Magazine

Lie on your back and bring your right knee in toward your chest. Hold onto your right thigh above your right knee and pull your knee over toward the left side of your body. Try to keep your right shoulder on the floor. If you can, look over your right shoulder. Repeat with the left leg.

Upper Back

While you're standing, clasp both hands together and gently pull away from your chest as you keep your back upright. Continue to clasp your hands as you raise your arms overhead.

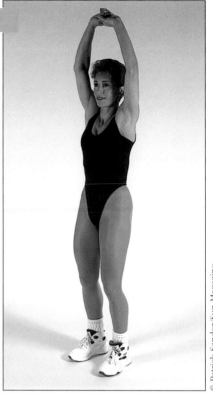

© Patrick Sandor/Sun Magazine

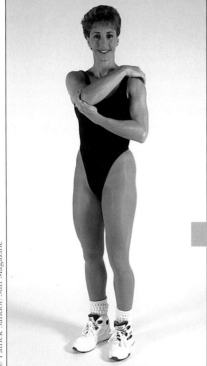

© Patrick Sandor/Sun Magazine

Shoulders and Triceps

Bring your right arm across your chest at shoulder level. Hold onto your arm above your elbow with your left hand and gently pull to the point of tension. Be sure to keep your right shoulder pressed down. Repeat with the left arm.

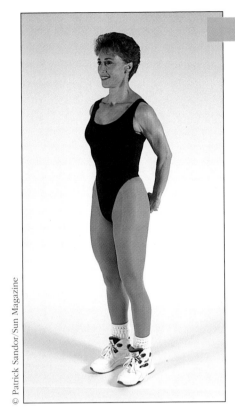

© Patrick Sandor/Sun Magazine

Front of Shoulders

Place both hands behind your back. If you can, clasp your hands and gently lift up to the point of tension. Maintain good posture as you do this stretch.

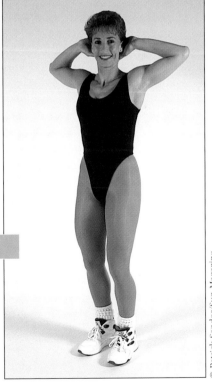

© Patrick Sandor/Sun Magazine

Chest

Place both hands behind your head. Open your elbows wide as if you are squeezing your elbows together behind you. You should feel your chest opening like a book.

Safe Stretching Tips

- Hold cool-down stretches for at least 30 to 60 seconds. Relax your body against any tension you may feel in the muscle or joint. The longer you hold the stretch position, the more you will increase muscle and joint flexibility.

- Try never to overstretch or to lock a joint. If you feel pain, stop. Pain is your body's natural warning mechanism that something is not right.

- Use deep cleansing breaths as you stretch. Hold a stretch to the point of tension, then take in a deep breath. As you exhale, let gravity help you to stretch closer to the ground. Repeat this process two to three times for each muscle group you are stretching to help increase your flexibility.

Finish each cool-down with a pat on the back or applause for a job well done!

PART II

AEROBICS WORKOUT ZONES

Now for the fun part—the workouts. The chapters in this part are organized into six color-coded workout zones. Each zone focuses on a specific length of time (duration) and intensity (how hard the workout feels). The workouts are distributed across the zones according to level of difficulty. Green workouts are the easiest. Blue workouts are a little more difficult, then Purple, Yellow, and Orange zones follow with increasing difficulty. The Red zone is the most challenging and advanced. Within each zone the workout difficulty also increases; the first workouts are the least demanding and the last workouts are the most challenging.

On each workout page you'll find everything you need to complete the workout: type of workout, duration, upper body and lower body movements listed on counts of the music, recommended music speed and style, estimated effort, suggested warm-up and cool-down, calories expended, and comments. In the next few sections I'll elaborate on some of those elements.

Intensity or Effort

Intensity is determined by heart rate or the rating of perceived exertion (RPE). The most challenging workouts are not only more physically demanding, but they also have more complex choreography.

Your intensity level can be determined in two different ways: with a heart rate check, or by checking how you feel throughout your workout. Do you feel strong, able to complete each combination, and able to talk? Or do you feel tired, unable to complete all of the combinations, or unable to talk as you work out? You should be able to talk and do your workout at the same time. If the intensity is too hard, it will be difficult to carry on a conversation and you should move to an easier workout zone.

As you work out, I encourage you to let your internal perception of effort be the guiding factor, not heart rate, speed of the music, or speed of the movement. Most aerobics enthusiasts do this. They know how easy or hard a workout is. Here, I've simply taken the next step and scored the degree of difficulty of each workout, and I'll ask you to do the same.

Dr. Gunnar Borg found that a person's sense of how difficult a workout feels lines up closely with objective measures of exertion, such as percentage of maximum heart rate. The Rating of Perceived Exertion (RPE) Scale, developed by Dr. Borg, can help you assess how hard you're working. On the 10-point scale, 0 is the feeling of no exertion at all, 1 is very light, 2 is light, 3 is moderate, 4 is somewhat heavy, 5 is heavy, 7 is very heavy, and 10 is very, very heavy (almost maximum).

WORKOUT COLOR ZONES			
Zone (chapter)	Type of workout	RPE/ % max HR	Time (min.)
Green (6)	Low intensity, short duration	1-3/55-69	10-25
Blue (7)	Low intensity, long duration	1-3/55-69	20-55
Purple (8)	Medium intensity, short duration	4-6/70-84	20-40
Yellow (9)	Medium intensity, long duration	4-6/70-84	30-55
Orange (10)	High intensity, short duration	7-10/85-100	12-35
Red (11)	High intensity, long duration	7-10/85-100	30-50

For reference, I've listed the approximate percentage of maximum heart rate that corresponds with each RPE level. The easiest way to determine your maximum heart rate is to subtract your age from 220:

Max heart rate = 220 − your age

If you're 25 years old, your maximum heart rate is about 195 BPM. If you're 40 years old, your maximum heart rate is about 180 BPM.

RPE scores of 1 to 3 for the Green and Blue workouts have corresponding heart rates of 55 percent to 69 percent of the maximum. The Purple and Yellow zone scores of 4 to 6 have corresponding heart rates of 70 percent to 84 percent of the maximum. Scores of 7 to 10 in the Orange and Red zones have corresponding heart rates of 85 percent to 100 percent of the maximum.

Caloric Cost

Doing aerobics is a fabulous way to burn calories and fat because many muscles are recruited from the upper body and lower body. The more muscles that you recruit during aerobics, the more kilocalories are burned. The table below is based on the workout zones and their respective aerobics activities.

Estimated Caloric Costs of Aerobics Exercises				
Zone	Aerobics activity	Kcal/min	Workout duration	Total
Green	Chair	2	<15	<30
	LIA	3	<25	<90
	Step	4	<20	<100
Blue	Chair	2	>20	>60
	LIA	3	>20	>90
	Step	4	>20	>120
Purple	LIA	6	<40	<180
	Hi/Lo	6	<40	<180
	Step	8	<40	<240
Yellow	LIA	6	>30	>170
	Hi/Lo	6	>35	>200
	Step	8	>30	>220
Orange	Hi/Lo	10	<20	<260
	Interval	12	<35	<360
	Step	15	<35	<400
	Slide	20	<35	<600
Red	Hi/Lo	10	>30	>350
	Interval	12	>30	>400
	Step	15	>35	>500
	Slide	20	>30	>600

It's difficult to precisely determine caloric consumption for a specific individual, but we can give estimates. Estimates are based on a 130-pound person. Add 10 percent to these totals for each 15 pounds over 130, and subtract 10 percent for each 15 pounds under 130. For example, in a Blue workout where an average of four kilocalories per minute are burned over a 30-minute period, a 130-pound woman would burn approximately 120 kilocalories:

$$4 \text{ kcal/min} \times 30 \text{ minutes} = 120 \text{ kcal}$$

A 145-pound woman who does the same workout would burn 132 kilocalories:

$$120 \text{ kcal} + (.10 \times 120 \text{ kcal}) = 132 \text{ kcal}$$

Beats Per Minute (BPM)

Each workout gives a suggested beats per minute range. Recall from chapter 2 that beats per minute indicate the speed of the music. Because aerobics coordinates music with movements, the speed of the music can also determine intensity, range of motion of movement, and overall energy.

Each workout has suggested music that works well with the style and intensity of the particular aerobics moves. For example, the BPM for step aerobics are slower (118 to 126) than hi/lo aerobics (135 to 158). When you step onto and off of a step according to the beats of the music, the slow tempo or speed allows you to execute your moves safely. Hi/lo aerobics moves work best when you move to a beat that is faster than step music.

You must feel comfortable and in control as you move to the music's beat. Use slower aerobics music if that feels better for you.

I take a "cookbook" approach to aerobics fitness training in the remainder of this book. In cooking, you achieve fabulous results by combining quality ingredients for proven recipes. The same is true here. First, I'll introduce the remaining ingredients by describing them completely through dozens of workouts in part II. Use the table on page 55 to familiarize yourself with the terminology used in the workouts. In part III I'll give you recipes for successful aerobics training according to your specific tastes and level of conditioning. Enjoy your aerobics workouts!

Aerobics Terminology

R	Right
L	Left
C	Center
OTS	On the spot, or in-place
Repeater	Successive repetition of the same move with the same foot or leg
3 peater	Repetition of the same move three times with the same foot or leg
4 peater	Repetition of the same move four times with the same foot or leg
S	Single
D	Double; indicates the same move is to be done two times
Alternate	Perform the move on one side, then the other; for example, with one arm then the other
Opposite	Move performed on the opposite side of the body; for example, R arm with L leg or L arm with R leg
Travel	The direction in which your entire body moves. *Knee lift travel forward*, for example, involves stepping forward after you place your foot on the floor after your knee lift. You can also travel backward, to either wall, or to the corner.
Lead	The foot or leg that starts a movement

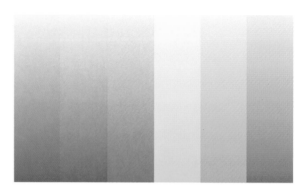

6

Green Zone

Green zone workouts are your easiest workouts. They are the lowest in intensity, with a perceived exertion rating between 1 and 3. They have a short duration, lasting less than 25 minutes.

The six Green zone workouts are adaptable to all levels of conditioning and ability. They are ideal for people who are just beginning their fitness program, for women who have recovered from labor and delivery, maturing adults, people with balance or coordination problems, or people with physical disabilities.

The Green workouts include chair aerobics, low impact aerobics (LIA), and step aerobics. The Green step combinations are easy to do. They can also be used as the cool-down portion of the more challenging Orange and Red zone workouts. Notice that all step workouts list the recommended height of the step and the starting position (lead).

If you've never tried any of the styles of Green zone workouts before, take your time. Don't let yourself feel frustrated; it's normal to go through a learning curve. Your most important assignment is to have fun!

TOTAL TIME: 20-25 minutes

WARM-UP: Chair warm-up

MUSIC SPEED AND STYLE: 120-130 BPM
"Club Trax 2," side A
"Stay on Track Step Reebok #8," side A

EFFORT: RPE 1-2

1

WORKOUT

Counts	Lower body	Upper body
1-8	Stationary in chair	Biceps curl × 8
9-16	Stationary in chair	Upright row × 16
17-64	Repeat × 3 more sets	
1-8	Stationary in chair	Lateral deltoid raise × 8
9-16	Stationary in chair	Chest press × 8
17-64	Repeat × 3 more sets	
1-8	Stationary in chair	Small circles × 8
9-16	Stationary in chair	Press down × 8
17-64	Repeat × 3 more sets	

1

2

3

TIME: Link combinations 1, 2, and 3 for 10-15 minutes.

COOL-DOWN: Chair cool-down

CALORIES EXPENDED: 20-30

COMMENTS

The exercises involve different shoulder angles. If you have any shoulder discomfort, stop and modify your moves so your arms stay down below shoulder level.

2

TOTAL TIME: 20-25 minutes

WARM-UP: Hi/lo warm-up

MUSIC SPEED AND STYLE: 120-130 BPM
  "Cardio Country 2," side B
  "Motown Step 2," side A

EFFORT: RPE 1-2

WORKOUT

1

2

3

Counts	Lower body	Upper body
1-8	March forward × 8	Pump × 8
9-16	Step touch (OTS) × 4	Biceps curl × 4
17-24	March backward × 8	Pump × 8
25-32	Step touch (OTS) × 4	Biceps curl × 4
33-128	Repeat × 3 more sets	
1-32	Touch step (side) × 16	Lateral deltoid raise × 16
1-8	Triplet (travel R) × 4	Sway low × 4
9-16	Twist (back to center) × 8	Sway low × 8
17-24	Triplet (travel L) × 4	Sway low × 4
25-32	Twist (back to center) × 8	Sway low × 8

TIME: Link combinations 1, 2, and 3 for 10-15 minutes.

COOL-DOWN: Hi/lo cool-down

CALORIES EXPENDED: 40-70

COMMENTS

Do the biceps curl as you do the touch of the step touch in combination 1. This is a great workout for all levels. The music and movements may seem slow, but this is an opportunity for you to make your moves be as big as you can without momentum doing the work for you. Enjoy!

LIA WORKOUT

TOTAL TIME: 25-30 minutes

WARM-UP: Hi/lo warm-up

MUSIC SPEED AND STYLE: 125-135 BPM
 "Mid-Tempo Mix 1," side B
 "Slide Reebok," side A

EFFORT: RPE 2

3

WORKOUT

Counts	Lower body	Upper body
1-8	Grapevine R, step touch × 2	Press down × 3, clap × 2
9-16	Grapevine L, step touch × 2	Press down × 3, clap × 2
17-64	Repeat × 3 more sets	
1-8	Skip × 8	Circles low at side × 8
9-16	Touch step front × 4	Pull back low × 4
17-64	Repeat × 3 more sets	
1-5	Knee lift (R, L, R) × 3	Chest press × 3
6-8	March (R, L, R) × 3	Punch down × 3
9-13	Knee lift (L, R, L) × 3	Chest press × 3
14-16	March (L, R, L) × 3	Punch down × 3
17-64	Repeat × 3 more sets	

TIME: Link combinations 1, 2, and 3 for 15-20 minutes.

COOL-DOWN: Hi/lo cool-down

CALORIES EXPENDED: 50-80

COMMENTS

In combination 2, pretend that you're skipping rope. Simulate the same arm movements as you skip. Make the touch step front in combination 2 a little "funky" if you'd like. Move your hips up and down, forward and back as you do this move. Just have fun!

4

TOTAL TIME: 30-35 minutes

WARM-UP: Hi/lo warm-up

MUSIC SPEED AND STYLE: 130-140 BPM
"Mid-Tempo Power Mix 1," side A

EFFORT: RPE 2-3

WORKOUT

Counts	Lower body	Upper body
1-8	Touch step side (travel forward) × 4	Lateral deltoid raise × 4
9-16	March back × 8	Pump × 8
17-64	Repeat × 3 more sets	
1-16	Low kick forward × 8	Punch up × 8
17-32	Slide-slide-ball-change × 4	Overhead press × 4
33-128	Repeat × 3 more sets	
1-4	Walk forward × 3, tap	Press down × 3 and clap
5-8	Walk backward × 3, tap	Press down × 3 and clap
9-16	Step touch front × 4	Pull back low × 4
17-64	Repeat × 3 more sets	

1

2

3

TIME: Link combinations 1, 2, and 3 for 20-25 minutes.

COOL-DOWN: Hi/lo cool-down

CALORIES EXPENDED: 60-90

COMMENTS

If you have difficulty doing the slide-slide-ball-change with the overhead press, delete the arms. If you still have difficulty, do double step touch R and double step touch L.

STEP WORKOUT

TOTAL TIME: 20-25 minutes

WARM-UP: Step warm-up

EQUIPMENT AND LEAD: Step 6 inches high, lead from the floor

MUSIC SPEED AND STYLE: 118-120 BPM
"Motown Step," side A
"Stay on Track Step Reebok #8," side A

EFFORT: RPE 1-2

5

WORKOUT

	Counts	Lower body	Upper body
1	1-16	Basic R lead × 4, tap down	Biceps curl × 8
	17-32	Basic L lead × 4, tap down	Biceps curl × 8
	33-64	Repeat × 1 more set	
2	1-16	V Step (R lead) × 4	Lateral deltoid raise × 4
	17-32	V Step (L lead) × 4	Press down × 16
	33-64	Repeat × 1 more set	
3	1-32	Turn step × 8	Alternate press forward × 8

TIME: Link combinations 1, 2, and 3 for 10-15 minutes.

COOL-DOWN: Step cool-down

CALORIES EXPENDED: 60-90

COMMENTS

The combinations in this workout are very simple so you can get used to step training if you are new to it. Be sure to look at your step and correct your foot placement. If you're experienced, you can use the workout as a cool-down. Please note that "Stay on Track Step Reebok" is music that is appropriate for warming up but not appropriate for step training. Be sure to listen to your music and watch the beats per minute.

6

TOTAL TIME: 25-30 minutes

WARM-UP: Step warm-up

EQUIPMENT AND LEAD: Step 6 inches high, lead from the floor

MUSIC SPEED AND STYLE: 118-120 BPM
  "The Assembly Line Step Reebok #6," side A

EFFORT: RPE 2

WORKOUT

Counts	Lower body	Upper body
1 1-16	Alternate gluteal squeeze × 4	Front raise × 4
17-32	Alternate knee lift × 4	Alternate punch up × 4
33-128	Repeat × 3 more sets	
2 1-8	Abductor lift × 1, over the top	Lateral deltoid raise × 1
9-16	Abductor lift × 1, over the top	Lateral deltoid raise × 1
17-64	Repeat × 3 more sets	
3 1-12	Kick (R lead) × 3	Pump × 12
13-16	Turn step (R lead) × 1	Press R arm forward × 1
17-28	Kick (L lead) × 3	Pump × 12
29-32	Turn step (L lead) × 1	Press forward L arm × 1
33-128	Repeat × 3 more sets	

TIME: Link combinations 1, 2, and 3 for 15-20 minutes.

COOL-DOWN: Step cool-down

CALORIES EXPENDED: 70-100

COMMENTS

The combinations involve more than one type of movement. Be sure to keep your abdominals tight as you lift your leg or kick. Only lift your leg as far as you comfortably can in combinations 1 and 2, maintaining good posture and alignment. When you do the kicks in combination 3, lift your leg no higher than your opposite knee.

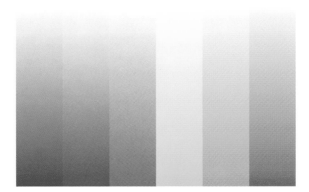

7

Blue Zone

Blue zone workouts offer the same types of workouts, effort, and benefits as the Green zone. They are rather light, with a perceived exertion rating of between 1 and 3. The major difference is in the length of each workout. The maximum workout duration in Blue workouts (55 minutes) is much longer than the maximum workout duration in the Green zone (25 minutes).

You should feel capable of doing each of the six Blue workouts, whether you're a novice or advanced aerobics enthusiast. Your present level of conditioning will determine if the longest workout in this chapter (65 minutes) feels good for you.

Some of the workout combinations may seem familiar to you, other combinations will be new. Workout 4 has a Latin theme. Enjoy each of these workouts and let the music and moves flow!

CHAIR WORKOUT

1

TOTAL TIME: 30-45 minutes

WARM-UP: Chair warm-up

MUSIC SPEED AND STYLE: 120-130 BPM
   "Broadway Step," side A
   "Resonant Energy Step Reebok #13," side A and B

EFFORT: RPE 1-2

WORKOUT

Counts	Lower body	Upper body
1-8	March	Lateral deltoid raise × 8
9-16	March	Triceps kickback × 8
17-64	Repeat × 3 more sets	
1-8	Hop (both feet)	Press down × 8
9-16	Hop (both feet)	Overhead press × 4
17-64	Repeat × 3 more sets	
1-32	Alternate knee lift × 16	Big circles × 16

TIME: Link combinations 1, 2, and 3 for 20-35 minutes.

COOL-DOWN: Chair cool-down

CALORIES EXPENDED: 60-90

COMMENTS

Your lower body can do whatever you feel most comfortable doing. If you prefer to keep your feet still, that's fine. However, if you choose to coordinate lower and upper body together, be sure to sit tall with good posture and alignment throughout the workout. Avoid slouching. Hold your abdominal muscles in and keep your chest lifted like an open window.

LIA WORKOUT

TOTAL TIME: 30-45 minutes

WARM-UP: Hi/lo warm-up

MUSIC SPEED AND STYLE: 120-130 BPM
  "Cardio Country 2," side B
  "Adding Horsepower Step Reebok #12," side B

EFFORT: RPE 1-2

WORKOUT

	Counts	Lower body	Upper body
1	1-8	March forward × 3, march back × 3	Small circles × 3
	9-16	March forward × 3, march back × 3	Small circles × 3
	17-32	Step touch (OTS) × 8	Clap × 8
	33-128	Repeat × 3 more sets	
2	1-4	Grapevine R	Lateral deltoid raise × 2
	5-8	Press up × 2	Overhead press × 2
	9-16	Reverse all (L lead)	
	17-64	Repeat × 3 more sets	
3	1-8	Alternate knee lift × 4	Alternate punch forward × 4
	9-16	Twist (back) × 8	Lateral triceps press × 8
	17-64	Repeat × 3 more sets	

TIME: Link combinations 1, 2, and 3 for 20-35 minutes.

COOL-DOWN: Hi/lo cool-down

CALORIES EXPENDED: 90-120

COMMENTS

When you do the press up in combination 2, be sure to use control, and squeeze your gluteal muscles without locking your knees. Then, as you come back down, bend your knees. This is a 2-count movement. Up on 1, down on 2. In combination 3, the alternate punch forward is opposite to the knee that lifts.

LIA WORKOUT

TOTAL TIME: 45-60 minutes

WARM-UP: Hi/lo warm-up

MUSIC SPEED AND STYLE: 125-135 BPM
"Mid-Tempo Power Mix 2," side B
"Slide Reebok," side A

EFFORT: RPE 2

3

WORKOUT

Counts	Lower body	Upper body
1-8	Step touch (travel forward) × 4	Clap × 4
9-12	March back × 4	Punch down × 4
13-16	Press up × 2	Overhead press × 2
17-32	Reverse all (L lead)	
33-128	Repeat × 3 more sets	
1-8	Alternate step touch rear (R lead) × 4	Front raise × 4
9-16	Double lunge (R and L)	Front raise × 4
17-24	Twist (OTS) × 8	Sway low × 8
25-32	Twist (OTS) × 8	Sway high × 8
33-64	Reverse all (L lead)	
65-128	Repeat × 1 more set	
1-8	Alternate knee lift (travel to R wall) × 4	Big circles × 4
9-16	Skip × 8, turn to face L wall	Small circles low at side × 8
17-24	Alternate knee lift (travel to L wall) × 4	Big circles × 4
25-32	Skip × 8, turn to face R wall	Small circles low at side × 8
33-128	Repeat × 3 more sets	

TIME: Link combinations 1, 2, and 3 for 35-50 minutes.

COOL-DOWN: Hi/lo cool-down

CALORIES EXPENDED: 100-130

COMMENTS

After you've finished linking all of your combinations, be sure to repeat the entire link again for the allotted workout time. At the end of combination 3, at the L wall, skip to face front to repeat the entire linked sequence.

As you step touch rear in combination 2, hold your abdominal muscles tight, and keep your chest lifted to avoid straining your back.

LIA WORKOUT

TOTAL TIME: 50-65 minutes

WARM-UP: LIA warm-up

MUSIC SPEED AND STYLE: 135-145 BPM
"Latin Power Mix," side A
"Musica Caliente," side A

EFFORT: RPE 2-3

4

WORKOUT

Counts	Lower body	Upper body
1-8	Triplet × 4	Sway low × 4
9-16	Twist (travel back to center) × 8	Sway low × 8
17-32	Reverse all (L lead)	
33-128	Repeat × 3 more sets	
1-8	Touch step (R lead) × 4	Press forward × 4
9-16	R touch 4 peater	Triceps kickback (R) × 4
17-32	Reverse all (L lead)	
33-128	Repeat × 3 more sets	
1-13	Mambo (R, diagonal to L corner) × 3-1/2	Front raise × 4
14-16	Cha-cha-cha	Clap × 3
17-32	Reverse all (L lead, diagonal to R corner)	
33-128	Repeat × 3 more sets	

1

2

3

TIME: Link combinations 1, 2, and 3 for 40-55 minutes.

COOL-DOWN: Hi/lo cool-down

CALORIES EXPENDED: 110-140

COMMENTS

Cha-cha-cha is a great transition to another lead foot. The rhythm of the move flows on 2 counts but uses the "and" beat in between. Cha (1)-cha (&)-cha (2).

The mambo move is where one foot steps forward (the other foot stays OTS) then steps back (the other foot stays OTS) for 4 counts. R forward (1), step L (2), R back (3), and step L (4). If you really want to "get into it," move your hips along with the rhythm of the music.

TOTAL TIME: 30-45 minutes

WARM-UP: Step warm-up

EQUIPMENT AND LEAD: Step 6 inches high, lead from the floor

MUSIC SPEED AND STYLE: 118-120 BPM
    "Step Power Mix #8," side A
    "The Assembly Line Step Reebok #6," side A

EFFORT: RPE 1-2

5

WORKOUT

	Counts	Lower body	Upper body
1	1-8	Basic R lead × 2	Punch up × 2, punch down × 2 for 2 sets
	9-16	V step (R) × 2	Lateral deltoid raise × 2
	17-24	V step (L) × 2	Lateral deltoid raise × 2
	25-32	Basic L lead × 2	Punch up × 2, punch down × 2 for 2 sets
	33-128	Repeat × 3 more sets	
2	1-12	Turn step, ball-change (R lead) × 3	Monkey × 12
	13-16	Abductor lift (L lead) × 1	Lateral deltoid raise (long lever) × 1
	17-28	Turn step, ball-change (L lead) × 3	Monkey × 12
	29-32	Abductor lift (R lead) × 1	Lateral deltoid raise (long lever) × 1
	33-128	Repeat × 3 more sets	
3	1-12	Knee lift × 1, gluteal squeeze × 1, knee lift × 1 (R lead)	Punch up × 1, biceps curl × 2, punch up × 1
	13-16	Corner to corner (R lead)	Small circles × 4
	17-28	Knee lift × 1, gluteal squeeze × 1, knee lift × 1 (L lead)	Punch up × 1, biceps curl × 2, punch up × 1
	29-32	Corner to corner (L lead)	Small circles × 4

STEP WORKOUT

TIME: Link combinations 1, 2, and 3 for 20-35 minutes.

COOL-DOWN: Step cool-down

CALORIES EXPENDED: 120-150

COMMENTS

Corner to corner is a fun way to go over the top of your step, on a diagonal. Remember that over the top is in 4 counts and follows with a tap down. Be sure to look at your step as you travel backward in combination 3.

STEP WORKOUT

TOTAL TIME: 45-60 minutes

WARM-UP: Step warm-up

EQUIPMENT AND LEAD: Step 6 inches high, lead from the floor

MUSIC SPEED AND STYLE: 118-120 BPM
"Step Power Mix #6," side B
"Stay on Track Step Reebok #8," side A

EFFORT: RPE 2

6

WORKOUT

	Counts	Lower body	Upper body
1	1-8	Alternate knee lift (R lead) × 2	Pull back low × 4
	9-16	3 peater knee lift, tap down (R lead)	Pump × 8
	17-24	A step × 2	Front raise × 4
	25-28	Turn step (R lead) × 1	Press R arm forward × 1
	29-32	Tap up (L lead) × 1	Clap × 2
	33-64	Reverse all (L lead)	
	65-128	Repeat × 1 more set	
2	1-12	Abductor lift (R lead) L end of step × 3	Lateral deltoid raise × 6
	13-16	Across the top (R lead) × 1	Big circles × 1
	17-32	Abductor lift (L lead) R end of step × 3	
	33-128	Repeat × 3 more sets	
3	1-8	L step (R lead) L end of step × 1	Pull down × 4
	9-16	L step (L lead) R end of step × 1	Pull down × 4
	33-128	Repeat × 3 more sets	

TIME: Link combinations 1, 2, and 3 for 35-50 minutes.

COOL-DOWN: Step cool-down

CALORIES EXPENDED: 130-160

COMMENTS

In combination 1, the claps are done as you tap up and tap down. If you don't feel comfortable doing across the top in combination 2, do grapevine on the floor behind your step.

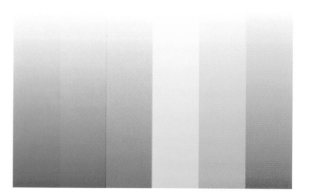

Purple Zone

Purple zone workouts are more intense and complex than the Blue and Green zone workouts. The workouts carry a perceived exertion rating of 4 to 6 and last 20 to 40 minutes.

The Purple zone uses three combinations of aerobics moves in a workout. However, the combinations involve more movement parts, so each of the combinations is a little more complex. For example, Blue workout 5, combination 3 and Purple workout 4, combination 2 both contain tap up and corner to corner moves, but the Purple workout adds an over the top move and more rapid transitions. This may seem like a small difference, but when you're moving in your combination to the music, you will feel the difference.

A great benefit of working in the Purple zone is that it's not too hard and not too easy. The workout should feel just right if your conditioning level is average to superior.

The Purple zone workouts include low impact aerobics (LIA) and step training in horizontal and vertical positions. In addition, the last few workouts are high and low impact aerobics (hi/lo) combinations. Workout 6 even uses Latin music and movements.

Fasten your seat belt and explore movement variations as you journey through Purple zone workouts.

TOTAL TIME: 35-45 minutes

WARM-UP: Hi/lo warm-up

MUSIC SPEED AND STYLE: 135-145 BPM
"Aerobics Power Mix #19," side B
"Disco Fever 1," side B

EFFORT: RPE 4

1

WORKOUT

Counts	Lower body	Upper body
1-4	Alternate touch step with heel (front) × 2	Alternate pull back high × 2
5-32	Repeat × 7 more sets	
1-8	Walk in circle R × 8	Small circles × 8
9-16	Press up × 4	Overhead press × 4
17-24	Walk in circle L × 8	Small circles × 8
25-32	Press up × 4	Overhead press × 4
33-128	Repeat × 3 more sets	
1-8	Twist (OTS) × 8	Monkey × 8
9-16	Alternate knee lift × 4	Alternate biceps curl × 8
17-32	Repeat all	
33-128	Repeat × 3 more sets	

TIME: Link combinations 1, 2, and 3 for 25-35 minutes.

COOL-DOWN: Hi/lo cool-down

CALORIES EXPENDED: 120-180

COMMENTS

Be sure to make your circle wide and large in combination 2. To protect your back in combination 3, execute your twists with your feet under your hips. When you do the overhead press, position your hands at a 45-degree angle toward the wall in front of you to help protect your shoulder joints.

LIA WORKOUT

TOTAL TIME: 40-50 minutes

WARM-UP: Hi/lo warm-up

MUSIC SPEED AND STYLE: 135-150 BPM
"Broadway Power Mix"
"Hi-Impact 19"

EFFORT: RPE 4-5

WORKOUT

Counts	Lower body	Upper body
1-8	Alternate hamstring curl (R lead, travel forward) × 4	Pull back low × 4
9-16	March back × 8	Pump × 8
17-64	Repeat × 3 more sets, facing all four walls	
1-8	Walk (travel to R wall) × 8	Small circles × 8
9-16	4 peater touch (R lead)	Lateral triceps press (R) × 4
17-24	Walk (travel to L wall) × 8	Small circles × 8
25-32	4 peater touch (L lead)	Lateral triceps press (L) × 4
1-4	Grapevine (R)	Overhead press × 2
5-8	Step touch × 2	Clap × 2
9-12	Grapevine (L)	Overhead press × 2
13-16	Step touch × 2	Clap × 2
17-64	Repeat × 3 more sets	

TIME: Link combinations 1, 2, and 3 for 30-40 minutes.

COOL-DOWN: Hi/lo cool-down

CALORIES EXPENDED: 140-180

COMMENTS

In combination 1, step with your right foot first, then curl your left hamstring. When you march back, your right foot will lead. In combination 2, the 4 peater touch is a transition move from one foot to the other.

STEP WORKOUT

TOTAL TIME: 30-40 minutes

WARM-UP: Step warm-up

EQUIPMENT AND LEAD: Step 8 inches high, lead from the floor

MUSIC SPEED AND STYLE: 120-122 BPM
  "Step Power Mix #8," side A
  "Step Reebok #12," side A

EFFORT: RPE 4-5

3

WORKOUT

Counts	Lower body	Upper body
1-8	Basic R lead × 2	Pull back low × 4
9-16	V step (R lead) × 2	Lateral deltoid raise × 4
17-24	Basic L lead × 2	Pull back low × 4
25-32	V step (L lead) × 2	Lateral deltoid raise × 4
33-128	Repeat × 3 more sets	
1-4	Turn step (R lead), tap down	Punch down × 4
5-8	Knee lift (L lead) × 1	Alternate punch forward × 4
9-12	Turn step (L lead), tap down	Punch down × 4
13-16	Knee lift (R lead) × 1	Alternate punch forward × 4
17-64	Repeat × 3 more sets	
1-4	Over the top (R lead)	Overhead press × 1
5-8	Over the top (L lead)	Overhead press × 1
9-32	Repeat × 3 more sets	

TIME: Link combinations 1, 2, and 3 for 20-30 minutes.

COOL-DOWN: Step cool-down

CALORIES EXPENDED: 180-220

COMMENTS

In combination 2, try to punch your arms with intensity; feel your arms as they move through space. If the intensity for over the top feels too difficult in combination 3, do a grapevine on the floor, passing the side of your step. Conversely, if you want to increase your intensity, you can add a little hop on top of your step as you transfer your weight.

TOTAL TIME: 35-45 minutes

4

WARM-UP: Step warm-up

EQUIPMENT AND LEAD: Step 8 inches high, lead from the floor

MUSIC SPEED AND STYLE: 120-122 BPM
  "Step Power Mix," side B
  "Adding Horsepower Step Reebok #12," side A

EFFORT: RPE 4-6

WORKOUT

Counts	Lower body	Upper body
1 1-16	Alternate knee lift × 4	Chest press × 8
17-32	Alternate gluteal squeeze × 4	Front raise × 8
33-128	Repeat × 3 more sets	
2 1-4	Corner to corner (R lead)	Small circles × 4
5-8	Over the top (L lead), tap down	Big circles × 1
9-12	Abductor lift (R lead) × 1, tap down	Lateral deltoid raise × 2
13-14	Face front, gluteal squeeze (R lead) × 1	Front raise × 1
15-16	Step down L foot, step down R foot	
17-32	Reverse all (L lead)	
33-128	Repeat × 3 more sets	
3	(Start this combination at the far R of your step, L foot steps up first.)	
1-12	Hamstring curl (L lead) × 3	Biceps curl × 6
13-16	Across the top	Sway high × 4
17-32	Reverse all (R lead) at the far L of your step	
33-128	Repeat × 3 more sets	

STEP WORKOUT

TIME: Link combinations 1, 2, and 3 for 25-35 minutes.

COOL-DOWN: Step cool-down

CALORIES EXPENDED: 200-240

COMMENTS

The alternate knee lift in combination 1 can travel from one side of the step to the other. For example, when your right foot leads, place your right foot on the left corner closest to you. When you do this, your body will naturally turn slightly toward the L wall. Do the reverse when the L foot leads. When you're linking your combinations at the end of combination 2, instead of transferring your feet, simply continue to let your left foot lead so that you can begin combination 3 at the right side of your step. If you feel the intensity in combination 3 is too difficult for you, simply do a grapevine on the floor instead of traveling across the entire step.

TOTAL TIME: 40-50 minutes

WARM-UP: Step warm-up

EQUIPMENT AND LEAD: Step 8-10 inches high, vertical position, lead from the top

MUSIC SPEED AND STYLE: 122-124 BPM
"Step Power Mix #6," side A
"Step Reebok Power Combinations II," side A

EFFORT: RPE 5-6

5

WORKOUT

Counts	Lower body	Upper body
1-8	Straddle down (R lead) × 2	Pull back low × 4
9-16	Lunge (R, L, double R)	Biceps curl × 4
17-24	Straddle down (L lead) × 2	Pull back low × 4
25-32	Lunge (L, R, double L)	Biceps curl × 4
33-128	Repeat × 3 more sets	
1-8	Squat down (R side) × 4	Hands on thighs to support back
9-16	Squat down (L side) × 4	Hands on thighs to support back
17-64	Repeat × 3 more sets	
1-8	Straddle down (R lead), alternate knee lift (travel forward) × 2	Opposite punch up × 2
9-16	Straddle down (R lead), alternate knee lift (travel back) × 2	Opposite punch up × 2
17-28	Basic R lead (off the end) × 3	Circles low at side × 12
29-32	Step down (off the end) × 2, knee lift (L) × 1	Circles low × 2, punch up (R) × 1
33-64	Reverse all (L lead)	
65-128	Repeat × 1 more set	

STEP WORKOUT

TIME: Link combinations 1, 2, and 3 for 30-40 minutes.

COOL-DOWN: Step cool-down

CALORIES EXPENDED: 200-240

COMMENTS

This workout may feel different if you're not used to doing step aerobics leading from the top. Use these helpful hints: (1) Always step off your step by stepping back, then step forward as you step onto your step. (2) Squats should be done with your legs slightly turned out from your hip. Be sure that your knees stay over your toes and your back stays straight. (3) Keep your heel off of the floor with lunges. Squeeze through your gluteal muscles, and keep your supportive knee facing the narrow end of your step. (4) In combination 2, quickly transfer from one side of your step to the other. In combination 3, be sure to look down at your step when you are traveling back to the end. Your knee lift at the end of your step is to help you switch to the opposite lead foot.

HI/LO WORKOUT

TOTAL TIME: 30-40 minutes

WARM-UP: Hi/lo warm-up

MUSIC SPEED AND STYLE: 136-142 BPM
"Latin Power Mix," side A
"Musica Caliente," side A

EFFORT: RPE 4-5

6

WORKOUT

Counts	Lower body	Upper body
1-8	Triplet (travel forward) × 4	Sway low × 4
9-12	March back × 4	Punch down × 4
13-14	Jack (out, in, out)	Lateral deltoid raise × 2
15-16	Hold feet out	Clap 1-2-3
17-32	Reverse all (L lead)	
33-64	Repeat × 1 more set	
1-2	Mambo (R lead) × 1	Press down × 1
3-4	Cha-cha-cha (R, L, R)	Front raise × 1
5-8	Mambo (L lead) × 1, cha-cha-cha (L, R, L)	Press down × 1, front raise × 1
9-32	Repeat × 3 more sets	
1-8	Jog to R wall × 8	Overhead press and clap × 4
9-12	Touch step front (R) × 1, touch step front (L) × 1	Biceps curl (R) × 1, biceps curl (L) × 1
13-16	Shuffle (travel R) × 4	Pull back low × 4
17-32	Reverse all (L lead)	
33-128	Repeat × 3 more sets	

TIME: Link combinations 1, 2, and 3 for 20-30 minutes.

COOL-DOWN: Hi/lo cool-down

CALORIES EXPENDED: 140-180

COMMENTS

If you prefer not to do moves with rhythmic variations, you can modify them. Do step touch instead of the mambo, or just step (step, step, step) instead of the cha-cha-cha.

HI/LO WORKOUT

TOTAL TIME: 35-45 minutes

WARM-UP: Hi/lo warm-up

MUSIC SPEED AND STYLE: 135-145 BPM
"Aerobics Power Mix #18," side B
"Performance Hi #16," side A

EFFORT: RPE 4-6

7

WORKOUT

	Counts	Lower body	Upper body
1	1-8	Jog forward × 8	Overhead press and clap × 4
	9-16	Step touch (back) × 4	Clap × 4
	17-24	Twist (OTS) × 8	Sway high × 8
	25-32	Twist (OTS) × 8	Sway low × 8
	33-64	Reverse all (L lead)	
	65-128	Repeat × 1 more set	
2	1-4	Grapevine (R lead, travel R), knee lift (L, turn to face rear)	Clap × 1
	5-8	Grapevine (L lead, facing rear), knee lift (R)	Clap × 1
	9-12	Grapevine (R lead, travel R, facing rear), knee lift (L, turn to face front)	Clap × 1
	13-16	Grapevine (L lead, facing front), knee lift (R)	Clap × 1
	17-64	Repeat × 3 more sets	

3

Counts	Lower body	Upper body
1-8	Lunge hop forward (R lead) × 4	Clap × 4
9-16	Squat (R), squat (L)	Biceps curl (R) with R squat, biceps curl (L) with L squat
17-24	Hop backward × 8	Press down × 8
25-32	Press up × 4	Overhead press × 4
33-64	Reverse all (L lead)	
65-128	Repeat × 1 more set	

TIME: Link combinations 1, 2, and 3 for 25-35 minutes.

COOL-DOWN: Hi/lo cool-down

CALORIES EXPENDED: 150-180

COMMENTS

In combination 2, clap as you lift your knee. The press up × 4 in combination 3 can be modified to a high impact jump, or you can do a mix of MIA and jumps: 3 MIA + 1 jump, 2 MIA + 2 jumps.

HI/LO WORKOUT

TOTAL TIME: 40-50 minutes

WARM-UP: Hi/lo warm-up

MUSIC SPEED AND STYLE: 140-155 BPM
"Aerobics Power Mix #19," side A
"Hi-Impact 15," side A

EFFORT: RPE 5-6

WORKOUT

Counts	Lower body	Upper body
1-8	Alternate knee lift (R lead) × 4, travel forward on R diagonal	Chest press × 4
9-12	March back × 4	Clap × 4
13-16	Jack × 2	Lateral deltoid raise × 2
17-32	Reverse all (L lead) on diagonal	
33-64	Repeat × 1 more set	
1-8	Split × 8	Alternate press forward × 8
9-12	March × 4	Punch down × 4
13-16	Knee lift (MIA) × 2	Overhead press × 2
17-32	Reverse all (L lead)	
33-64	Repeat × 1 more set	
1-8	Press up × 4	Overhead press × 4
9-16	Walk in circle R (R lead) × 8	Small circles × 8
17-32	Reverse all (L lead)	
33-64	Repeat × 1 more set	

TIME: Link combinations 1, 2, and 3 for 30-40 minutes.

COOL-DOWN: Hi/lo cool-down

CALORIES EXPENDED: 160-180

COMMENTS

In combination 3, you have the option of doing the press up as all MIA, mix the impact, or execute all of these as high impact with a jump. If you feel you'd like to increase the intensity even more, you can perform power moves where the knees pull in close to your chest as you jump very high.

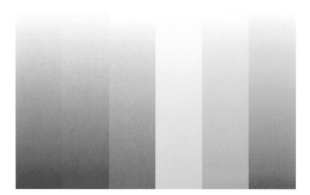

Yellow Zone

The Yellow zone takes the Purple zone workouts a step further. The Yellow zone workouts have an RPE rating between 4 and 6. Even though the intensity level is neither too easy nor too hard, the workouts are longer. The Yellows involve linking four combinations, they last more than 30 minutes, and they involve slightly more complex choreography. Workout 6 has a Broadway theme.

Some of the combinations are similar to those you learned in previous zones, and some new combinations are introduced. The Yellow zone is ideal for fitness enthusiasts of all levels of conditioning who prefer an aerobics workout that's longer than 30 minutes.

Enjoy the Yellow zone workouts; they are similar to the average intensity aerobics you'll find being done in a health club or studio.

TOTAL TIME: 40-50 minutes

WARM-UP: Hi/lo warm-up

MUSIC SPEED AND STYLE: 135-145 BPM
  "Aerobics Power Mix #20," side B
  "Disco Fever," side A

EFFORT: RPE 4

WORKOUT

Counts	Lower body	Upper body
1-8	Alternate knee lift (R lead) × 4	Alternate biceps curl × 8
9-16	Walk in circle R × 8	Small circles × 8
17-24	March forward (R lead) × 3, march back (L lead) × 3	Pump × 8
25-32	4 peater touch (R lead)	Triceps kickback × 4
33-64	Reverse all (L lead)	
65-128	Repeat × 1 more set	
1-8	Skip (OTS) × 8	Tap × 2, clap × 2, tap × 2, clap × 2
9-16	Step touch × 4	Open and cross × 4
17-32	Repeat all (L lead)	
33-128	Repeat × 3 more sets	
1-4	March to R front corner × 3	Press R arm to R corner × 2
5-8	March to L front corner × 3	Press L arm to L corner × 2
9-12	March to R back corner × 3	Press R arm to R corner × 2
13-16	March to L back corner × 3	Press L arm to L corner × 2
17-64	Repeat × 3 more sets	
1-8	V step (R lead) × 2	Lateral deltoid raise × 4
9-16	Press up × 4	Overhead press × 4
17-32	Reverse all (L lead)	
33-128	Repeat × 3 more sets	

TIME: Link combinations 1, 2, 3, and 4 for 30-40 minutes.

COOL-DOWN: Hi/lo cool-down

CALORIES EXPENDED: 170-220

COMMENTS

The 4 peater is a lateral touch that is repeated four times with the same leg. It's a great way to move from one foot leading to the other. When you do the press up in combination 4, be sure to extend your legs without jumping. The arms simply follow what the lower body is doing. You need to bend your elbows as you bend your knees.

TOTAL TIME: 50-60 minutes

WARM-UP: Hi/lo warm-up

MUSIC SPEED AND STYLE: 135-150 BPM
"70's Workout," side A
"Motown," side A

EFFORT: RPE 4-5

WORKOUT

Counts	Lower body	Upper body
1-4	Walk (R) × 3, tap L foot (to R wall)	Pump × 4
5-8	L foot touch (rear) × 2	Front raise × 2
9-16	Lunge (R) × 1, lunge (L) × 1, lunge (R) × 2	Punch forward × 4
17-32	Reverse all (L lead)	
33-128	Repeat × 3 more sets	
1-8	Triplet (travel forward) × 4	Sway low × 4
9-16	Alternate knee (OTS) × 4	Big circles × 4
17-24	Triplet (travel back) × 4	Sway low × 4
25-32	Alternate knee (OTS) × 4	Big circles × 4
33-128	Repeat × 3 more sets	
1-8	Skip (OTS) × 8	Monkey × 8
9-16	Twist (OTS) × 8	Lateral deltoid raise × 4
17-24	Alternate hamstring curl × 4	Biceps curl × 4
25-32	Double hamstring curl × 2	Biceps curl × 4
33-128	Repeat × 3 more sets	

4

Counts	Lower body	Upper body
1-4	Slide-slide-ball-change (R lead)	Overhead press × 1
5-8	Ball-change side and back (L foot)	Circles low at side × 4
9-12	March forward (L lead) × 3, tap	Pump × 3 and clap
13-16	March back (R lead) × 3, tap	Pump × 3 and clap
17-32	Reverse all (L lead)	
33-128	Repeat × 3 more sets	

TIME: Link combinations 1, 2, 3, and 4 for 40-50 minutes.

COOL-DOWN: Hi/lo cool-down

CALORIES EXPENDED: 180-240

COMMENTS

In combination 4, you'll do two extra ball-changes, placing the foot to the side of the body, then behind your R leg again. If you feel more comfortable doing slide-slide-ball-change with only one ball change, that's fine, but that is only 4 counts. You can add a slide-slide-ball-change to the L to equal 8 counts.

STEP WORKOUT

TOTAL TIME: 40-50 minutes

WARM-UP: Step warm-up

EQUIPMENT AND LEAD: Step 8 inches high, lead from the floor

MUSIC SPEED AND STYLE: 120-122 BPM
"Best of Step, Volume 1," side A
"Adding Horsepower Step Reebok #12," side A

EFFORT: RPE 4-5

3

WORKOUT

Counts	Lower body	Upper body
1-8	Basic R lead × 2	Chest press × 4
9-16	Grapevine (R and L)	Lateral deltoid raise × 4
17-28	Alternate knee lift (R, L, R) × 3	Alternate punch up × 3
29-32	Basic L lead × 1	Pump × 4
33-64	Reverse all (L lead)	
65-128	Repeat × 1 more set	
1-12	Turn step with ball-change (R, L, R) × 3	Punch down × 3, press up × 3
13-16	Abductor lift (L lead) × 1	Lateral triceps press × 1
17-32	Reverse all (L lead)	
33-128	Repeat × 3 more sets	
1-12	Knee lift × 1, abductor lift × 1, curl × 1 (R lead, travel backward)	Punch up × 1, lateral deltoid raise × 1, biceps curl × 1
13-16	Corner to corner	Small circles × 4
17-32	Reverse all (L lead)	
33-128	Repeat × 3 more sets	

4

Counts	Lower body	Upper body
1-8	Abductor lift at L end of step (R lead) × 2	Lateral triceps press × 2
9-16	Basic R lead (travel R) × 2	Overhead press × 2
17-32	Across the top × 4	Big circles × 4

TIME: Link combinations 1, 2, 3, and 4 for 30-40 minutes.

COOL-DOWN: Step cool-down

CALORIES EXPENDED: 220-260

COMMENTS

The alternate punch up in combination 1 is done as the knee lifts. The press up in the first part of combination 2 is done as the feet ball-change. Be sure to work at your own level of comfort.

TOTAL TIME: 45-55 minutes

WARM-UP: Step warm-up

EQUIPMENT AND LEAD: Step 8 inches high, lead from the floor

MUSIC SPEED AND STYLE: 120-122 BPM
   "Step Power Mix," side B
   "Resonant Energy," side A

EFFORT: RPE 4-6

WORKOUT

Counts	Lower body	Upper body
1-4	Basic R lead, cha-cha-cha	Pump × 5
5-8	Basic L lead, cha-cha-cha	Pump × 5
9-16	Straddle down, R 1/4 turn (face R wall)	Overhead press × 4
	Straddle down, R 1/4 turn (face the rear)	
17-32	Repeat facing rear (R lead)	Repeat upper body
33-56	Alternate knee lift (facing front) × 6	Pull down × 12
57-64	3 peater knee lift (R lead)	Monkey × 8
65-128	Reverse all (L lead)	
129-256	Repeat × 1 more set	
1-16	Kick (R lead, face L wall) × 4	Alternate punch forward × 16
17-20	March on the floor × 4	Punch down × 4
21-24	R cha-cha-cha (on top) to L corner, step down, step down behind step	Pump × 3, clap × 2
25-28	L cha-cha-cha (on top) to R corner, step down, step down behind step	Pump × 3, clap × 2
29-32	R cha-cha-cha (on top), step down, step down	Pump × 3, clap × 2
33-64	Reverse all (L lead)	
65-128	Repeat × 1 more set	

Counts	Lower body	Upper body
1-8	Basic R lead × 2	Open and cross × 4
9-12	V step (R) × 1	Press R arm up, L arm up, R arm down, L arm down
13-16	Jack (on the floor) × 2	Lateral deltoid raise × 2
17-32	Reverse all (L lead)	
33-128	Repeat × 3 more sets	
1-16	Alternate knee lift (R lead) × 4, travel around the entire step	Alternate punch up × 4
17-24	Gluteal squeeze (R) × 1, gluteal squeeze (L) × 1	Monkey × 4
25-32	3 peater gluteal squeeze (R lead)	Monkey × 8
33-64	Reverse all (L lead)	

TIME: Link combinations 1, 2, 3, and 4 for 35-45 minutes.

COOL-DOWN: Step cool-down

CALORIES EXPENDED: 240-280

COMMENTS

Each combination uses great transitional moves. The first combination transitions from one foot lead to another with a step-ball-change. If this is too difficult, simply tap down. The second also uses a rhythmic cha-cha-cha on the top of the step to switch from one foot to another. The third uses a jack on the floor and the last combination uses a 3 peater. The alternate knee lift during which you travel around the entire step is also called *around the world*. After you do the R lead knee lift facing the L wall, straddle your step and continue to face the L wall with the L lead. Then turn to face the R wall to repeat R lead knee lift, straddle the step, and continue to face the R wall with L lead knee lift. The arm punches up as you lift your knee. The 1/4 turns in combination 1 should always be done with your feet turned out, so turn toward the R wall with the R lead.

STEP WORKOUT

TOTAL TIME: 50-60 minutes

WARM-UP: Step warm-up

EQUIPMENT AND LEAD: Step 8-10 inches high, vertical position, lead from the floor

MUSIC SPEED AND STYLE: 122-124 BPM
"Step Power Mix #6," side B
"Adding Horsepower Step Reebok #12," side A

EFFORT: RPE 5-6

WORKOUT

Counts	Lower body	Upper body
1-8	T step at end of step (R lead)	Alternate lateral triceps press × 8
9-16	Grapevine (R), grapevine (L) on floor	Alternate biceps curl × 8
17-32	Reverse all (L lead)	
33-128	Repeat × 3 more sets	
1-8	Abductor lift (R lead) L side of step × 2	Lateral deltoid raise × 2
9-12	Over the top × 1	Small circles × 4
13-16	March around front of step × 4, face rear	Press L arm forward × 1
17-32	Reverse all (L lead)	
33-128	Repeat × 3 more sets	
	(Stand astride the step.)	
1-8	Alternate knee lift (travel forward) × 2	Punch up × 2
9-16	3 peater knee lift (R lead)	Open and cross × 3
17-32	Reverse all (L lead, travel back)	
33-128	Repeat × 3 more sets	

4

Counts	Lower body	Upper body
1-8	Step up and squat (to L side), squat (to R side) (both feet end up on top of the step)	Biceps curl (L), biceps curl (R)
9-16	Straddle down (L lead) × 2	Pull down × 4
17-32	Reverse all (R lead)	
33-128	Repeat × 3 more sets	

TIME: Link combinations 1, 2, 3, and 4 for 40-50 minutes.

COOL-DOWN: Step cool-down

CALORIES EXPENDED: 250-300

COMMENTS

Remember that "astride your step" means to stand with the step between your legs. A squat is a great transition move to get you from floor lead to top lead and top lead back down to floor lead. Do squats to transition back down to floor lead so you can begin to link with combination 1, which leads from the floor.

TOTAL TIME: 45-60 minutes

WARM-UP: Hi/lo warm-up

MUSIC SPEED AND STYLE: 130-140 BPM
"Broadway Power Mix," side A

EFFORT: RPE 4-5

6

WORKOUT

Counts	Lower body	Upper body
1-8	Triplet (travel R) × 4	Sway low × 4
9-12	March (OTS) × 4	Punch down × 4
13-16	Jack × 2	Lateral deltoid raise × 2
17-32	Reverse all (L lead)	
33-64	Repeat × 3 more sets	
1-5	Alternate knee lift (R lead) × 3	Alternate punch forward × 3
6-8	3 steps	Small circles × 3
9-16	Reverse all (L lead)	
17-64	Repeat × 3 more sets	
1-4	Slide-slide-ball-change	Open and cross × 1
5-8	Ball-change × 2 (1 side, 1 rear)	Open and cross × 1
9-16	Kick × 4 (L, R, L, R)	Press forward × 4
17-32	Reverse all (L lead)	
33-128	Repeat × 3 more sets	

1 *2* *3*

4

Counts	Lower body	Upper body
1-8	Jog forward × 8	Overhead press and clap × 4
9-16	Jog in a circle × 8	Double punch up and down for 2 sets
17-24	Alternate heel press forward × 8, travel back	Alternate press forward × 8
25-32	Twist (OTS) × 8	Alternate lateral triceps press × 8
33-64	Reverse all (L lead)	
65-128	Repeat × 1 more set	

TIME: Link combinations 1, 2, 3, and 4 for 35-50 minutes.

COOL-DOWN: Hi/lo cool-down

CALORIES EXPENDED: 200-250

COMMENTS

These hi/lo combinations really mix the intensity and impact with a Broadway flair. Even if you don't have access to Broadway-style music, just kick up your feet as you pretend that you're in New York, New York!

TOTAL TIME: 50-60 minutes

WARM-UP: Hi/lo warm-up

MUSIC SPEED AND STYLE: 135-145 BPM
"Classic Rock Workout," side A
"Rockin' Aerobics," side A

EFFORT: RPE 4-6

WORKOUT

Counts	Lower body	Upper body
1-4	March forward (R lead) × 3, kick L	Small circles × 3 and clap
5-8	March back (L lead) × 3, kick R	Small circles × 3 and clap
9-16	Step touch rear (OTS) × 4	Open and cross × 4
17-24	Skip (OTS) × 8	Circles low at side × 8
25-32	Knee lift (L, R, L, R)	Big circles × 4
33-64	Reverse all (L lead)	
65-128	Repeat × 1 more set	
1-8	Kick side (R, L, R, L, travel forward) × 4	Alternate lateral triceps press × 8
9-16	Double jack × 2	Punch up × 2, clap 2 for 2 sets
17-24	Kick rear (travel back) × 4	Pull back × 4
25-32	Press up × 4	Overhead press × 4
33-64	Reverse all (L lead)	
65-128	Repeat × 1 more set	

Counts	Lower body	Upper body
1-8	Jog (R lead, travel to R wall) × 8	Pull back high × 4
9-12	Face R wall, touch lateral (S, S)	Lateral deltoid raise (long lever) × 2
13-16	Touch R foot (D)	Lateral deltoid raise (long lever) × 2
17-32	Reverse all (L lead)	
33-128	Repeat × 3 more sets	
1-8	Twist (travel R) × 8	Monkey × 8
9-16	Alternate heel touch (L lead) × 4	Press down × 4
17-32	Reverse all (L lead)	
33-128	Repeat × 3 more sets	

TIME: Link combinations 1, 2, 3, and 4 for 40-50 minutes.

COOL-DOWN: Hi/lo cool-down

CALORIES EXPENDED: 230-280

COMMENTS

The alternate heel touch in combination 4 can be done as LIA, MIA, or HIA, depending on your level of conditioning. The feet remain on the floor with the LIA option, the supporting heel lifts with the MIA option, and the supporting foot jumps off the floor with the HIA option.

TOTAL TIME: 55-65 minutes

WARM-UP: Hi/lo warm-up

MUSIC SPEED AND STYLE: 140-155 BPM
"Aerobics Power Mix #19," side A
"Performance Hi+Lo Impact #12," side A

EFFORT: RPE 5-6

8

WORKOUT

Counts	Lower body	Upper body
1-8	Step touch (travel forward) × 4	Open and cross × 4
9-16	March back × 8	Double punch up and down for 2 sets
17-32	Lunge (S, S, D) × 2, finish facing R wall	Punch forward (R, L, then both)
33-64	Reverse all (L lead)	
65-128	Repeat × 1 more set	
1-8	Lunge hop (forward to L wall) × 4	Clap × 4
9-16	Split × 8	Alternate press forward × 8
17-24	LIA hamstring curl × 4	Biceps curl × 4
25-32	Twist (travel back to face front) × 8	Alternate biceps curl × 8
33-64	Reverse all (L lead to R wall)	
65-128	Repeat × 1 more set	
1-8	Double grapevine (travel R)	Punch down × 3 and clap for 2 sets
9-16	Double grapevine (travel L)	Punch down × 3 and clap for 2 sets
17-32	V step (L lead) × 4	Lateral deltoid raise × 8
33-64	Reverse all (L lead)	
65-128	Repeat × 1 more set	

4

Counts	Lower body	Upper body
1-4	Jog forward × 4	Overhead press and clap × 2
5-8	Slide (travel R) × 4	Small circles × 4
9-12	Jog backward × 4	Overhead press and clap × 2
13-16	Slide (travel L) × 4	Small circles × 4
17-24	Alternate knee lift × 4	Big circles × 4
25-32	Jack × 4	Lateral deltoid raise × 4
33-64	Reverse all (L lead)	
65-128	Repeat × 1 more set	

TIME: Link combinations 1, 2, 3, and 4 for 45-55 minutes.

COOL-DOWN: Hi/lo cool-down

CALORIES EXPENDED: 250-300

COMMENTS

The lunges in the first combination will help you change the direction you'll face for the next combination. The slide is a moderately intense move. If you prefer to modify it, do double grapevine traveling both directions. The jog and slide in combination 4 will form a box as you travel.

10

Orange Zone

The Orange zone workouts take you into the advanced aerobics enthusiast category. These workouts are physically and mentally challenging and may take you out of your comfort zone with moves and combinations you may never have experienced before. Consult chapter 4 for descriptions of any of the new moves in this zone.

The rating of perceived exertion for the Orange workouts is from 7 to 10 (the maximum). The duration is 35 minutes or less. The primary focus is to increase not only intensity, but also the complexity and variety of the moves and combinations. Four combinations of moves are done in each workout.

The Orange zone introduces two new forms of aerobics: interval training and slide training. *Interval training* is high intensity aerobics activity that alternates with low intensity activity. The high intensity activity is hi/lo aerobics, which may also incorporate power moves. The low intensity activity (called *active recovery*) can be anything from non-impact aerobics to muscle conditioning with resistance apparatus to a light walk. The muscle conditioning intervals are given as "MC" in the workouts. *Slide training* is high intensity lateral training that involves a slide board with rubber bumpers on either end. It requires some technical skill and an advanced fitness level.

Some of the Orange step workouts incorporate power step moves. Power step moves are advanced moves that are similar to traditional aerobic power moves in that they make your body lift high off the ground by forcing the legs to push hard off the floor or your step.

HI/LO WORKOUT

TOTAL TIME: 22-30 minutes

WARM-UP: Hi/lo warm-up

MUSIC SPEED AND STYLE: 135-145 BPM
 "Cardio Country," side A
 "Disco Fever" side B

EFFORT: RPE 7-8

WORKOUT

Counts	Lower body	Upper body
1-8	Alternate knee lift (travel forward, R lead) × 4	Chest press × 4
9-16	Walk in circle R × 8	Pump × 8
17-32	Squat (R, C, L, C) × 2	Pull down × 8
33-64	Reverse all (L lead)	
65-128	Repeat × 1 more set	
1-12	Grapevine (R, L, R, travel forward)	Press R arm forward × 2, Press L arm forward × 2, Press R arm forward × 2
13-16	Hop back × 4	Pull back low × 4
17-28	Grapevine (L, R, L, travel forward)	Press L arm forward × 2, Press R arm forward × 2, Press L arm forward × 2
29-32	Hop back × 4	Pull back low × 4
1-8	Jog forward × 4, slide R × 4 small circles × 4	Overhead press and clap × 2,
9-16	Jog back × 4, slide L × 4 small circles × 4	Overhead press and clap × 2,
17-24	Alternate hamstring curl × 4	Biceps curl × 4
25-32	4 peater hamstring curl (R lead)	Monkey × 8
33-64	Reverse all (L lead)	
65-128	Repeat × 1 more set	

Counts	Lower body	Upper body
1-8	Mambo R toward L wall × 2	Pump × 8
9-12	Jack × 2	Lateral deltoid raise × 2
13-16	Press up × 2	Overhead press × 2
17-32	Reverse all (L lead)	
33-128	Repeat × 3 more sets	

TIME: Link combinations 1, 2, 3, and 4 for 12-20 minutes.

COOL-DOWN: Hi/lo cool-down

CALORIES EXPENDED: 210-260

COMMENTS

The LIA and HIA moves are all mixed up in this workout to give you maximum benefit with minimum stress to your joints. If you prefer not to jump, simply do the moves as low impact. For example, jacks can be modified to be touch step × 2.

INTERVAL WORKOUT

TOTAL TIME: 22-30 minutes

WARM-UP: Hi/lo warm-up

MUSIC SPEED AND STYLE:
Hi/lo = 145-150 BPM; "Aerobics Power Mix #19," side A
MC = 120-130 BPM; "Resonant Energy," side A

EFFORT: RPE 7-8

WORKOUT

Counts	Lower body	Upper body
1-8	Alternate knee lift (travel forward) × 4	Opposite arm punch (forward) × 4
9-12	Walk in circle R × 4	Pump × 4
13-16	Hop (facing front) × 4	Clap × 4
17-32	Reverse all (L lead)	
33-36	Grapevine (R)	Small circles × 3 and clap
37-40	Press up × 1, power jump × 1	Overhead press × 2
41-44	Grapevine (L)	Small circles × 3 and clap
45-48	Press up × 1, power jump × 1	Overhead press × 2
49-64	Repeat grapevine combo (R and L)	
65-128	Repeat × 1 more set	
1-2 min.	Upright row with tubes or bands	
1-8	Jog forward (R lead) × 8	Overhead press and clap × 4
9-16	Split × 3 and hold, split × 3 and hold	Opposite press forward × 3 and hold
17-24	March back × 8	Punch up and down × 4
25-32	Jack (OTS) × 4	Lateral deltoid raise × 4
33-64	Reverse all (L lead)	
65-128	Repeat × 1 more set	
1-2 min.	Row and triceps kickback. R leg back in a calf stretch, one end of tube placed under L foot, R arm holds other end of tube. Lift elbow to the ceiling, extend forearm to the rear, bend the elbow, then lower down (8 counts). Work each arm for 1 minute.	

	Counts	Lower body	Upper body
3	1-16	Alternate kicks (S, S, D; S, S, D; R lead)	Front raise × 8
	17-24	Twist (travel R) × 8	Sway high × 8
	25-32	Twist (travel L) × 8	Sway low × 8
	33-64	Reverse all (L lead)	
	65-128	Repeat × 1 more set	
MC	1-2 min.	Squats with or without weights	
4	1-8	Slide (R) × 3, 1/2 turn (face rear), slide (L) × 3	Punch down × 3, clap on 1/2 turn, punch down × 3
	9-16	Slide (R) × 3, 1/2 turn (face front), slide (R) × 3	Punch down × 3, clap on 1/2 turn, punch down × 3
	17-32	V step (R lead) × 4	Punch up × 2, down × 2 for 4 sets
	33-64	Reverse all (L lead)	
	65-128	Repeat × 1 more set	
MC	1-2 min.	Biceps curls with weights, tubes, or bands	

TIME: Link combinations 1, 2, 3, and 4 for 12-20 minutes.

COOL-DOWN: Hi/lo cool-down

CALORIES EXPENDED: 230-300

COMMENTS

Interval training is one of the most efficient ways to burn fat. The secret is to switch very quickly from the high intensity activity to the low intensity recovery and back to the high intensity activity. Don't let your body recover completely. Try to push yourself during the aerobic phase so that there is a noticeable difference in intensity during the active recovery phase.

TOTAL TIME: 35-45 minutes

WARM-UP: Hi/lo warm-up

MUSIC SPEED AND STYLE:
Hi/lo = 145-158 BPM; "Performance Hi+Lo Impact #17," side A
MC = 110-120 BPM; "Hip Hop Funk," side B

EFFORT: RPE 8-9

WORKOUT

Counts	Lower body	Upper body
1-8	Alternate knee lift (R lead) × 4	Opposite arm punch up × 4
9-12	March wide × 4	Pump × 4
13-16	Jack (in, out, in, hold)	Cross, open, cross
17-24	Skip (OTS) × 8	Biceps curl × 8
25-32	Step touch (L lead) × 4	Lateral deltoid raise (long lever) × 4
33-64	Reverse all (L lead)	
65-128	Repeat × 1 more set	
1-2 min.	Lateral deltoid raise with opposite lateral leg lift. Work each arm and leg for 1 minute.	
1-8	Double grapevine (R)	Punch down × 3 and clap for 2 sets
9-16	Power slide (travel L) × 4	Upright row × 4
17-24	V step (L lead) × 2	Small circles × 8
25-32	Press up × 2, power jump × 2	Overhead press × 4
33-64	Reverse all (L lead)	
65-128	Repeat × 1 more set	
1-2 min.	Pull back high with bands or weights while doing squats.	

3

Counts	Lower body	Upper body
1-8	Jog (toward R wall) × 8	Overhead press and clap × 4
9-16	4 peater knee lift (R), face front	Triceps kickback (R arm) × 4
17-24	Kick (rear, L lead) × 4	Pull back low × 4
25-32	Jog forward × 4, jack × 2	Clap × 4, big circles × 2
33-64	Reverse all (L lead to L wall)	
65-128	Repeat × 1 more set	

MC

1-2 min.	Lunge (R) × 8, lunge (L) × 8. Repeat for allotted time.	

4

Counts	Lower body	Upper body
1-8	Lunge hop (forward, R lead) × 4	Clap × 4
9-16	Hop (back) × 8	Punch down × 8
17-32	Reverse all (L lead)	
33-128	Repeat × 3 more sets	

MC

1-2 min.	With elbows pressed into sides, rotate forearm to the side then back to center to work the rotator cuff muscles.

TIME: Link combinations 1, 2, 3, and 4 for 25-35 minutes.

COOL-DOWN: Hi/lo cool-down

CALORIES EXPENDED: 260-360

COMMENTS

In MC interval 1, working the opposing leg with the opposing arm will help with your balance. You'll be working the abductors of the lower body and the shoulder of the upper body. In MC interval 3, be sure to place your knee under your hip as you do your lunges. Squeeze your buttocks together as you straighten your legs. Keep your hands on your thighs to support your back and move at a pace that is comfortable for you. Remember, slower is better. In combination 1, *march wide* is a march with your feet wider.

4

TOTAL TIME: 30-40 minutes

WARM-UP: Step warm-up

EQUIPMENT AND LEAD: Step 8-10 inches high, lead from the floor

MUSIC SPEED AND STYLE: 122-124 BPM
"Cardio Power Mix 1," side B
"Resonant Energy," side A

EFFORT: RPE 7-8

WORKOUT

Counts	Lower body	Upper body
1		
1-4	Basic R lead × 1	R arm up, L arm up, clap, pull down
5-8	V step (R lead) × 1	Clasped hands over R shoulder, over L shoulder
9-12	Basic R lead × 1	Punch up × 2, clap × 2
13-16	Knee lift (R lead)	Punch up (R) × 1
17-32	Reverse all (L lead)	
33-128	Repeat × 3 more sets	
2		
1-4	Turn step (R lead) × 1	Press R arm forward × 1
5-8	Power knee lift (L lead) × 1	Punch up (L) × 1
9-16	A step (L lead) × 2	Front raise × 4
17-32	Reverse all (L lead)	
33-128	Repeat × 3 more sets	
3		
1-12	Kick (R lead) × 3	Alternate punch forward × 12
13-16	March on floor × 4	Punch down × 4
17-32	Alternate power tap up (R lead) × 4	Clap × 4 with tap
33-64	Reverse all (L lead)	
65-128	Repeat × 1 more set	

4

Counts	Lower body	Upper body
1-12	Basic R lead × 3	Pull back low × 6
13-16	Power V step (on top) × 1, jack together × 1, hold for 2 counts	Punch up, clap, small circles × 2
17-24	Lunge rear single (R lead, from the top) × 4	Triceps kickback × 4
25-28	Lunge rear double (R lead) × 1	Triceps kickback × 2
29-32	Lunge rear (L lead), knee lift, step down (L and R)	Triceps kickback × 1
33-64	Reverse all (L lead)	
65-128	Repeat × 1 more set	

TIME: Link combinations 1, 2, 3, and 4 for 20-30 minutes.

COOL-DOWN: Step cool-down

CALORIES EXPENDED: 250-350

COMMENTS

The power options for some of these basic moves are an advanced option. If you prefer not to jump, that's fine. Do what you feel most comfortable doing. The advanced option to the basic × 2 R lead in combination 1 is run step × 2 or power leap on count 2. The power V in combination 4 is a jump up onto your step with the legs out (count 1), then jack in together (count 2), then hold for 2 counts (counts 3 and 4). Remember that power moves require you to jump from the floor to the top of your step in a single bound.

STEP WORKOUT

5

TOTAL TIME: 35-45 minutes

WARM-UP: Step warm-up

EQUIPMENT AND LEAD: Step 8 inches high, lead from the floor

MUSIC SPEED AND STYLE: 122-126 BPM
"Motown Step 2," side A
"Increasing Your RPM's Step Reebok #10," side A

EFFORT: RPE 8-10

WORKOUT

	Counts	Lower body	Upper body
1	1-8	Alternate knee lift (R lead) × 2	Alternate punch up × 2
	9-16	3 peater knee lift (R lead)	Monkey × 6
	17-28	Over the top (R lead) × 3	Overhead press × 3
	29-32	Power kick (L lead) × 1	Clap × 1
	33-64	Reverse all (L lead)	
	65-128	Repeat × 1 more set	
2	1-12	Turn step, ball-change (R lead) × 3	Punch down × 3, punch up × 1 for 3 sets
	13-16	Power abductor leap (L lead) × 1	Lateral deltoid raise × 1
	17-32	Reverse all (L lead)	
	33-128	Repeat × 3 more sets	
3	1-4	Kick (R lead) × 1	Clap × 2
	5-8	Power tap up (R lead) × 1	Overhead press × 1
	9-12	Power over the top (R lead) × 1	Small circles × 4
	13-16	Walk around to back of step (L lead) × 4	Press L arm forward × 1
	17-32	Reverse all (L lead)	
	33-128	Repeat × 3 more sets	

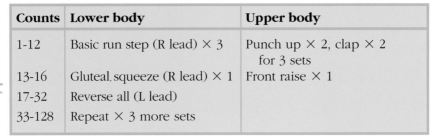

4

Counts	Lower body	Upper body
1-12	Basic run step (R lead) × 3	Punch up × 2, clap × 2 for 3 sets
13-16	Gluteal squeeze (R lead) × 1	Front raise × 1
17-32	Reverse all (L lead)	
33-128	Repeat × 3 more sets	

TIME: Link combinations 1, 2, 3, and 4 for 25-35 minutes.

COOL-DOWN: Step cool-down

CALORIES EXPENDED: 300-400

COMMENTS

Remember to look down at your step while you do these advanced step combinations.

SLIDE WORKOUT

TOTAL TIME: 30-40 minutes

WARM-UP: Slide warm-up

MUSIC SPEED AND STYLE: 120-126 BPM
"Lynne Brick Power Mix," side B
"The Assembly Line Step Reebok #6," side A

EFFORT: RPE 8-9

WORKOUT

Counts	Lower body	Upper body
1-32	Basic slide × 4 strokes	Open and cross × 4
1-4	Slide squat (R lead)	Overhead press × 1, front raise with squat
5-8	Knee lift (L) and squat	Pull back L arm high with knee lift, then front raise with squat
9-16	Reverse all (L lead)	
17-64	Repeat × 3 more sets	
1-4	Basic slide (R lead)	Press up, clap, and pull down × 1
5-8	Lunge (L) × 2	Small circles × 2
9-16	Reverse all (L lead)	
17-64	Repeat × 3 more sets	
1-8	Cross country slide (fast, R lead, facing L wall) × 8	Opposite arm press forward × 8
9-14	Cross country (slow) × 3	Punch up × 2, punch down × 2 for 3 sets
15-16	Slide feet together, 1/2 turn to opposite wall	Arms at sides
17-32	Reverse all (L lead, facing R wall)	
33-128	Repeat × 3 more sets	

TIME: Link combinations 1, 2, 3, and 4 for 20-30 minutes.

COOL-DOWN: Slide cool-down

CALORIES EXPENDED: 400-500

COMMENTS

Remember to evert your feet as you approach the bumper and to place your feet up onto your bumper, or deceleration ramp. Keep your knees over your toes, chest lifted, and eyes focused forward. If you're not ready for slide combinations, continue to practice the basic slide until you feel comfortable with the movement and your body placement. Remember to keep one foot placed on the bumper as you do any variation of moves such as lunges, taps, squats, and so on.

The cross country slide in combination 4 can be done close to your bumper (if you're concerned about your balance) or away from your bumper in the center of your slide.

TOTAL TIME: 35-45 minutes

WARM-UP: Slide warm-up

MUSIC SPEED AND STYLE: 122-130 BPM
"Step Power Mix #9," side A
"Slide Reebok," side A

EFFORT: RPE 8-10

WORKOUT

Counts	Lower body	Upper body
1-16	Basic slide, double tap front (R lead) × 4	Open and cross, punch down together for 4 sets
17-32	Slide, tap rear (R lead) × 4	Open and cross, triceps kickback with tap rear for 4 sets
33-64	Repeat × 1 more set	
1-8	Diagonal lunge (R lead to R wall) × 2	Front raise × 2
9-16	Adductor slide (fast) × 4	Small circles × 4
17-24	Stationary skating stride (slow, R lead) × 4	Lateral triceps press (slow) × 4
25-32	Stationary skating (fast) × 8	Sway low × 8
33-64	Reverse all (L lead)	
65-128	Repeat × 1 more set (travel to the L bumper on the last 4 quick skates)	
1-8	Athletic slide (low profile, R lead) × 4	Opposite arm press forward × 4
9-16	Basic slide (R lead) × 2	Clap as foot lands on bumper × 2
17-64	Repeat × 3 more sets	

4

Counts	Lower body	Upper body
1-4	Telemark (R lead, face R wall)	Front raise × 1
5-8	Squat (off R), return to center	Hands on thighs
9-12	Squat (off L), return to center	Hands on thighs
13-16	Twist (to face L wall)	Lateral triceps press × 4
17-32	Reverse all (L lead)	

TIME: Link combinations 1, 2, 3, and 4 for 25-35 minutes.

COOL-DOWN: Slide cool-down

CALORIES EXPENDED: 500-600

COMMENTS

Keep your body low and slide for 2 counts as you do your athletic slides (low profile) in combination 3.

11

Red Zone

The Red zone workouts require the highest level of aerobics activity. They have an RPE rating of 7 to 10, last longer than 30 minutes, and utilize five physically intense, complex workout combinations.

Once you've mastered the Reds, you are probably a candidate for other options in the fitness industry such as entering aerobics competitions or becoming certified and teaching fitness classes.

Have a great time as you journey through the Red zone workouts. Even if it takes you a long time to master the Reds, never give up. Challenging yourself physically and mentally will make attaining your goals that much more enjoyable.

HI/LO WORKOUT

TOTAL TIME: 40-50 minutes

WARM-UP: Hi/lo warm-up

MUSIC SPEED AND STYLE: 135-150 BPM
"Club Trax 1," side A
"Performance Hi+Lo Impact #17," side A

EFFORT: RPE 7-8

WORKOUT

Counts	Lower body	Upper body
1-8	Alternate heel tap (forward) × 4	Open and cross × 4
9-16	Alternate lunge (rear) × 4	Front raise × 4
17-64	Repeat × 3 more sets	
1-8	Lunge hop (travel forward, R lead) × 4	Clap × 4
9-16	V step (R lead) × 2	Punch up × 2, punch down × 2 for 2 sets
17-28	Kick rear (R lead) × 6	Pull back low as leg extends back × 6
29-32	Hop × 4	Clap 1-2, 1-2-3
33-64	Reverse all (L lead)	
65-128	Repeat × 1 more set	
1-8	Grapevine (R lead), grapevine (L lead)	R arm circle × 4, L arm circle × 4
9-12	Press up × 2	Press R arm up, press L arm up
13-16	Power jump × 1, hold × 2	Overhead press × 1, clap × 2
17-32	Reverse all (L lead)	
33-128	Repeat × 3 more sets	
1-8	Alternate lunge rear (R lead) × 4	Triceps kickback × 4
9-16	4 peater lunge (R lead, face the L wall)	Lateral triceps press R arm × 4
17-24	Jog (to L wall) × 8	Overhead press and clap × 4
25-32	Jack (to face front) × 4	Lateral deltoid raise × 4
33-64	Reverse all (L lead to R wall)	
65-128	Repeat × 1 more set	

1

5

Counts	Lower body	Upper body
1-4	Touch step (front, R lead) × 2	Opposite biceps curl × 2
5-8	Shuffle (R) × 4	Pull back low × 4
9-16	Double knee lift (L), double knee lift (R)	Chest press × 4
17-32	Reverse all (L lead)	
33-128	Repeat × 3 more sets	

TIME: Link combinations 1, 2, 3, 4, and 5 for 30-40 minutes.

COOL-DOWN: Hi/lo cool-down

CALORIES EXPENDED: 350-400

COMMENTS

Combination 5 is fun, simple, and incorporates rhythmic variations. The touch step is done in front. The ball-changes in the shuffle use the "and" beat of the music. Now because the weight of your body is on your R foot, you can do double knee lift L lead.

HI/LO WORKOUT

TOTAL TIME: 50-60 minutes

WARM-UP: Hi/lo warm-up

MUSIC SPEED AND STYLE: 145-158 BPM
  "Aerobics Power Mix #20," side A
  "Performance Hi+Lo Impact #17," side A

EFFORT: RPE 7-9

2

1

WORKOUT

Counts	Lower body	Upper body
1-8	March forward (R lead) × 8	Punch up and down for 4 sets
9-16	Slide-slide-ball-change (R lead, L lead)	Overhead press × 2
17-24	Repeat slide-slide-ball-change (R and L)	Overhead press × 2
25-32	Hop back × 8	Tap × 2, clap × 2 for 2 sets
33-64	Reverse all (L lead)	
65-128	Repeat × 1 more set	
1-3	Jog forward (R, L, R)	Pump × 3
4-8	Lateral kick (side) × 3	Alternate lateral triceps press × 6
9-11	Jog back (L, R, L)	Pump × 3
12-16	Lateral kick (side) × 3	Alternate lateral triceps press × 6
17-64	Repeat × 3 more sets	
1-8	Alternate knee (travel to R front corner) × 4	Opposite arm punch up × 4
9-16	Skip (OTS) × 8	Circles low at side × 8
17-24	Twist (travel back) × 8	Monkey × 8
25-32	Jack (facing front) × 4	Big circles × 4
33-64	Reverse all (L lead)	
65-128	Repeat × 1 more set	

1

2

3

	Counts	Lower body	Upper body
	1-4	Jog forward × 4	Overhead press and clap × 2
	5-8	Hop and turn to face rear × 4	R arm press forward
	9-12	Jog forward × 4	Overhead press and clap × 2
	13-16	Hop and turn to face front × 4	Press L arm forward
4	17-20	Squat (R) × 2	Pull back high × 2
	21-24	Feet together, squat down, power jump up, squat down	Pull down × 1, front raise with jump × 1, pull down × 1
	25-32	Reverse the squat sequence (L)	Pull back high × 2, pull down × 1, front raise × 1, pull down × 1
	33-64	Reverse all (L lead)	
	65-128	Repeat × 1 more set	
	1-8	Mambo (R lead, facing L wall) × 2	Pump × 7 and clap
	9-16	Mambo (L lead, facing R wall) × 2	Pump × 7 and clap
5	17-24	4 peater knee lift (HIA, L lead, facing R wall)	L arm pulls back high × 4
	25-32	Power jack × 2	Open and cross × 2
	33-64	Reverse all (L lead, start facing R wall)	
	65-128	Repeat × 1 more set	

TIME: Link combinations 1, 2, 3, 4, and 5 for 40-50 minutes.

COOL-DOWN: Hi/lo cool-down

CALORIES EXPENDED: 400-450

COMMENTS

Be sure to bend your knee as you march in combination 1. Think of making your whole body march, instead of just your feet. Power jacks in combination 5 require that you jump high off the floor. You'll do only 2 repetitions within 8 counts. If your prefer not to do power jacks, simply do 4 regular jacks or 4 alternate side toe touches.

INTERVAL WORKOUT

TOTAL TIME: 40-45 minutes

WARM-UP: Hi/lo warm-up

MUSIC SPEED AND STYLE:
Hi/lo = 135-150 BPM; "Club Trax 5, Tribal Beats," side A
MC = 118-122 BPM; "Power Toning," side A

EFFORT: RPE 7-8

3

WORKOUT

	Counts	Lower body	Upper body
1	1-8	Step touch (R lead) × 4	Overhead press × 4
	9-24	Grapevine (R and L) for 2 sets	Small circles × 3 and clap for 4 sets
	25-32	Twist (OTS) × 8	Sway high × 4, low × 4
	33-64	Reverse all (L lead)	
	65-128	Repeat × 1 more set	
MC	1-2 min.	Slow squat (down × 2 counts, up × 2 counts)	
2	1-8	Lunge hop (travel forward, R lead) × 4	Clap × 4
	9-16	Double knee lift (R and L)	Punch up, punch down × 4
	17-28	Kick rear (R lead) × 6	Pull back low × 6
	29-32	Jack (OTS) × 2	Big circles × 2
	33-64	Reverse all (L lead)	
	65-128	Repeat × 1 more set	
MC	1-2 min.	March with pull back high.	
3	1-8	3 steps forward, travel diagonally to R front corner, 3 steps to L corner	Press R arm to R corner × 2 and clap, press L arm to L corner × 2 and clap
	9-16	Jog back × 8	Pump × 8
	17-24	Step touch × 4	Clap × 4
	25-28	Press up × 2	Punch R arm up, L arm up
	29-32	Power jump × 1, hold × 2	Both arms up with power jump, clap × 2 with hold
	33-64	Reverse all (L lead)	
	65-128	Repeat × 1 more set	

INTERVAL WORKOUT

	Counts	Lower body	Upper body
MC	1-2 min.	Abductor lift with lateral deltoid raise (work R leg with L shoulder; L leg with R shoulder)	
4	1-8	Triplet (to R wall) × 4	Sway low × 4
	9-16	4 peater touch (R lead, turning to face front)	Triceps kickback × 4
	17-32	Reverse all (L lead to L wall)	
	33-128	Repeat × 3 more sets	
MC	1-2 min.	Triceps kickbacks with mambo. Work each arm for 1 minute.	
5	1-8	Power heel tap (front, R lead) × 4	Press down × 4
	9-16	Walk in circle R × 8	Pump × 8
	17-32	Reverse all (L lead)	
	33-128	Repeat × 3 more sets	
MC	1-2 min.	Lunges	

TIME: Link combinations 1, 2, 3, 4, and 5 for 30-35 minutes.

COOL-DOWN: Hi/lo cool-down

CALORIES EXPENDED: 400-500

COMMENTS

As you do any of the muscle conditioning active recovery, be sure to think about the muscle group you're working. The more you force the muscle or muscle group to contract, the more benefit you'll obtain. Work at a slow pace; slower is better so you can work through the entire range of motion without momentum doing the work for you. With squats or lunges, be sure to keep your knees over your toes, your abdominal muscles tight, and your back erect. Remember that with squats, your toes and heels are parallel to each leg but with lunges, one leg is forward with a bent knee and the other leg is back with a slightly bent knee placed under your hip. If you experience knee discomfort, externally rotate your legs out from the hip with squats and don't bend your knees as much in lunges.

TOTAL TIME: 50-60 minutes

WARM-UP: Hi/lo warm-up

MUSIC SPEED AND STYLE:
Hi/lo = 145-158 BPM; "Lynne Brick Power Mix," side A
MC = 122-126 BPM; "Lynne Brick Power Mix," side B

EFFORT: RPE 8-9

4

WORKOUT

	Counts	Lower body	Upper body
1	1-8	March back × 3, lift knee (R lead) for 2 sets	Punch down × 3, clap on knee lift
	9-16	Alternate step knee lift (travel forward) × 4	Sway low × 4
	17-32	1/2-time jack × 4 (out × 2, in × 2)	Open and cross × 4
	33-64	Reverse all (L lead)	
	65-128	Repeat × 1 more set	
MC	1-2 min.	Biceps curls with squats (add weights, bands, or tubes)	
2	1-8	V step (R lead) × 2	Lateral deltoid raise × 4
	9-24	Slide (R) × 3, slide (L) × 3 for 2 sets	Small circles × 3 and clap for 4 sets
	25-32	4 peater hamstring curl (R lead)	Monkey × 8
	33-64	Reverse all (L lead)	
	65-128	Repeat × 1 more set	
MC	1-2 min.	Squats (R, C, L, C)	
3	1-8	Kick forward (R lead) × 4	Front raise × 4
	9-16	Split (OTS) × 8	Alternate arm press forward × 8
	17-24	Twist (travel backward) × 8	Alternate biceps curl × 8
	25-32	Lunge (to the rear; S, S, D)	Triceps kickback × 4
	33-64	Reverse all (L lead)	
	65-128	Repeat × 1 more set	
MC	1-2 min.	Triceps kickbacks with heel presses in calf stretch position (add weights, bands, or tubes)	

Counts	Lower body	Upper body
1-8	Alternate touch to side (R lead, LIA) × 4	Lateral deltoid raise × 4
9-16	Power heel touch (front) × 4	Press down × 4
17-64	Repeat × 3 more sets	

4

MC | 1-2 min. | Abductor lifts slow × 4, fast × 8 | |

Counts	Lower body	Upper body
1-8	Power step touch × 4	Press up × 4
9-16	March (OTS) × 8	Punch down × 8
17-64	Repeat × 3 more sets	

5

MC | 1-2 min. | Upright rows with lunges (add weights, bands, or tubes) | |

TIME: Link combinations 1, 2, 3, 4, and 5 for 40-50 minutes.

COOL-DOWN: Hi/lo cool-down

CALORIES EXPENDED: 450-550

COMMENTS

Remember that with interval training you want to push yourself as hard as you can during the peak phases. Even if you don't feel comfortable jumping with the power moves, do each move as a low impact alternative with high intensity. The first combination, although relatively low impact, will make you move with the alternate step knee lifts forward. Feel as if you're skipping like a child.

STEP WORKOUT

TOTAL TIME: 45-60 minutes

WARM-UP: Step warm-up

EQUIPMENT AND LEAD: Step 6-8 inches high, lead from the floor

MUSIC SPEED AND STYLE: 122-126 BPM
   "Club Trax 6, Happy House Workout," side A
   "Adding Horsepower Step Reebok #12," side A

EFFORT: RPE 8-10

5

WORKOUT

	Counts	Lower body	Upper body
1	1-8	Basic R lead × 2	Tap × 2, clap × 2, open and cross × 4 (fast)
	9-12	Run step × 1	Punch up × 2, punch down × 2
	13-16	Knee lift (R lead) × 1	Punch up (R) × 1
	17-32	Reverse all (L lead)	
	33-128	Repeat × 3 more sets	
2	1-4	Power tap up (to L wall) × 1	Clap × 2
	5-8	Walk around to front side of step (facing R wall) × 4	Press R arm forward
	9-16	Power kick (R lead) × 2	Alternate punch forward × 8
	17-28	Turn step with ball-change × 3	Punch down × 3, punch up × 1 for 3 sets
	29-32	Power knee lift (L lead) × 1	Clap on knee
	33-64	Reverse all (L lead)	
	65-128	Repeat × 1 more set	

Counts	Lower body	Upper body
3		
1-8	U step (turn, straddle, turn)	Pull back low × 4 (R lead) × 1
9-16	Power abductor lift (L lead) × 2	Lateral triceps press × 2
17-24	March forward (on floor) × 3, march back × 3	Front raise × 2 and clap for 2 sets
25-32	Power over the top (L lead,	Overhead press × 2 R lead) × 2
33-64	Reverse all (L lead)	
65-128	Repeat × 1 more set	
4		
1-8	Basic run step (R lead) × 2	Punch up × 2, punch down × 2
9-12	V step × 1	R arm punch up, L arm punch up, both punch down × 2 (4 counts)
13-14	Jack × 1	Lateral deltoid raise × 1
15-16	Pull hips in × 2	Pull back low × 2
17-32	Reverse all (L lead)	
33-128	Repeat × 3 more sets	
5		
1-8	Kick forward (R lead) × 2	Alternate punch forward × 8
9-12	Over the top (R lead) × 1	Big circles × 1
13-16	Walk around to back side of	Small circles × 4 step (facing R wall)
17-32	Power knee lift (L lead) × 4	Overhead press × 4
33-64	Reverse all (L lead)	
65-128	Repeat × 1 more set	

TIME: Link combinations 1, 2, 3, 4, and 5 for 35-50 minutes.

COOL-DOWN: Step cool-down

CALORIES EXPENDED: 500-600

COMMENTS

The walk around the step in combinations 2 and 5 will enable you to face the opposite wall on the other side of the step. Remember that you don't have to do power step moves if you prefer not to jump. The move without the jump will not be as intense, but it may be just as effective.

SLIDE WORKOUT

6

TOTAL TIME: 40-50 minutes

WARM-UP: Slide warm-up

MUSIC SPEED AND STYLE: 120-126 BPM
  "Cardio Power Mix 2," side B
  "Slide Reebok"

EFFORT: RPE 8-9

WORKOUT

Counts	Lower body	Upper body
1-8	Basic slide, single knee lift (R and L)	Open and cross × 2
9-16	Basic slide, 3 peater lunge (L leg)	Punch L arm forward as leg lunges
17-32	Reverse all (L lead)	
33-128	Repeat × 3 more sets	
1-8	Cross country (travel back, facing L wall, L lead) × 8	Alternate press forward × 8
9-12	Telemark forward (R lead)	Front raise × 1
13-16	Lunge rear (R, facing L wall) × 1	Overhead press × 1
17-32	Reverse all (L lead, facing L wall)	
33-128	Repeat × 3 more sets	
1-8	Diagonal lunge (to L corner) × 2, travel to center	Front raise × 2
9-16	Stationary skating stride × 8	Alternate lateral triceps press × 8
17-32	Reverse all (R lead)	
33-128	Repeat × 3 more sets	

SLIDE WORKOUT

Counts	Lower body	Upper body
1-4	Corner to corner (R lead, toward R front corner)	Front raise × 1
5-10	Step off slide with L foot, 3 peater (R) abductor lift	Lateral deltoid raise × 3
11-12	Step onto slide (R foot, then L foot)	Hands on hips
13-16	Squat (on slide) × 2	Tap × 1, clap × 1 for 2 sets
17-32	Reverse all (L lead)	
33-128	Repeat × 3 more sets	
1-12	Adductor slide × 3	Open and cross × 3
13-16	Twist × 4	Sway low × 4
17-64	Repeat × 3 more sets	

TIME: Link combinations 1, 2, 3, 4, and 5 for 30-40 minutes.

COOL-DOWN: Slide cool-down

CALORIES EXPENDED: 600-700

COMMENTS

Look down at your slide board periodically to be sure that your feet are in correct placement. The diagonal lunge starts at the back end of the L side of your slide. Remember to place your L foot (your drag foot) against the bumper so you can easily push to the opposite corner. Leave some room between your feet to give you more balance. If you don't feel comfortable, modify the corner to corner to a basic slide. During the last set of twists in combination 5, travel toward your L bumper so you can begin the link of moves again.

SLIDE WORKOUT

TOTAL TIME: 45-55 minutes

WARM-UP: Slide warm-up

MUSIC SPEED AND STYLE: 122-126 BPM
"Club Trax 2, Techno Workout," side B
"Slide Reebok"

EFFORT: RPE 8-10

WORKOUT

	Counts	Lower body	Upper body
1	1-16	Basic slide, squat, knee lift, squat (R and L)	Overhead press × 1, front raise × 1, pull L arm back high × 1, front raise × 1 for 2 sets
	17-32	Basic slide and tap (rear) × 4	Open and cross, press down × 4
	33-128	Repeat × 3 more sets	
2	1-4	Telemark (R lead, face R wall)	Front raise × 1, biceps curl (R)
	5-8	Squat (off R), return to center	Biceps curl (R)
	9-12	Squat (off L), return to center	Biceps curl (L)
	13-16	Twist (to face R wall)	Sway high × 4
	17-32	Reverse all (L lead to L wall)	
	33-128	Repeat × 3 more sets (last twist turn to face L wall)	
3	1-8	Cross country (fast, travel back, R lead) × 8	Monkey × 8
	9-16	Basic slide (R and L) × 2	Open and cross × 2
	17-32	Athletic slide (low profile, R lead) × 8	Opposite arm press forward × 8
	33-128	Repeat × 3 more sets	

7

4

Counts	Lower body	Upper body
1-8	Athletic slide × 2, basic slide (R lead) × 1	Opposite arm press forward × 3
9-16	4 peater lunge lateral (L)	Press L arm forward × 4
17-32	Reverse all (L lead)	
33-128	Repeat × 3 more sets	

5

Counts	Lower body	Upper body
1-8	Adductor slide (slow) × 2	Lateral deltoid raise × 2
9-16	Adductor slide (fast) × 4	Small circles × 8
17-32	Adductor slide (very slow— 8 counts each) × 2	Open and cross × 2
33-128	Repeat × 3 more sets	

TIME: Link combinations 1, 2, 3, 4, and 5 for 35-45 minutes.

COOL-DOWN: Slide cool-down

CALORIES EXPENDED: 700-800

COMMENTS

Be sure to place your feet up onto your bumper each time you approach it, and especially when you're doing leg variations such as knee lifts and lunges. In combination 5, make the last slow adductor slide travel to your L bumper to begin the link of the combinations all over again. The most important thing is to have fun and let the movements flow into a rhythm. Flow and fun are the foundations of slide training. Enjoy!

PART III

TRAINING BY THE WORKOUT ZONES

Now that you've learned the ingredients in part II, you can create an exciting aerobics program that will lead to the results you want. Part III will help you do that. In the chapters that follow, you'll learn how the workouts can be organized into a training program. You'll also find sample programs and information about how to chart your progress.

Approaches to Aerobics

Your approach to aerobics will probably fit into one of the three categories that follow.

- **Beginning/easy aerobics.** You're a beginner if you've never participated in any aerobics programs, classes, or activities. You feel best doing the light or easy workouts. You'll probably accomplish your fitness goals doing three to four workouts per week.

- **Frequent/moderate aerobics.** As a frequent aerobics enthusiast, you train a little longer, faster, harder, and more often than a beginner. You qualify for this intensity level if you already participate in an aerobics program (e.g., at a health club or community center) or do any aerobic activity such as running, power walking, or cycling regularly four to five times per week. Your main workout goal is to improve your fitness.

  You prefer this level because you enjoy workouts that are a little more demanding than the beginning/easy workouts, yet not as physically and psychologically challenging as intense workouts. You favor workouts in which the impact forces on the lower body are moderate.

- **Competitive/intense aerobics.** Your emphasis is to set high personal fitness goals for your body and mind. You complete five or six workouts per week and enjoy doing physically challenging, high intensity workouts. You also enjoy the challenge of taxing your mind with complex aerobics routines.

The workout program you select depends largely on your aerobics activity preferences, current level of conditioning, and fitness goals. You'll soon discover which workouts work best for you, whether you follow a sample program like the ones I've provided or whether you put the workouts together on your own. There are dozens of workouts to choose from, so the possibilities are plentiful. Remember, no matter what your fitness level or goals, each workout should leave you feeling good on the inside and on the outside of your body. Let's take a look at how to put the workouts together.

12

Setting Up
Your Program

Challenge is motivational, and it is necessary for improvement. However, you must be physically and psychologically ready to handle the challenges of workouts that are beyond your comfort zone. You don't have to "kill yourself" to get a great aerobics workout. You'll probably get the most enjoyment out of aerobics if you choose your workouts based on what you can and want to do. The training guidelines that follow are for people of all fitness levels, fitness goals, ages, and experiences. They will help you pick workouts that are right for you.

Listen to Your Body

If you train your body at a level that is too easy, you won't make any fitness gains. If you train at levels that are too hard, you can become injured or ill or perform poorly. But training at levels that are just right will condition your body to adapt and improve. The more you condition your body, the more efficiently your body will perform. To find the right level, you'll need to understand what is too easy, too hard, or just right for your workouts. Your body will tell you what it can or can't handle, but you have to listen. The problem is that people often don't know what to listen for and how to respond.

The most important indicators of appropriate training are your heart rate, body weight, hours slept, and overall energy. If your resting heart rate is too high when you wake up in the morning, you have not completely recovered from the previous day's workout. If your body weight goes down too fast (more than one or two pounds per week), you're not adequately hydrating or nourishing yourself. If you don't get enough sleep, you'll find every workout, regardless of intensity level, a struggle. Your overall energy level should be heightened during and after each workout. If you feel too fatigued, you may be working too hard.

How can you tell if your body is adapting to your workout? Here's a checklist to help you listen to your body each morning:

1. Was your resting heart rate, taken just before stepping out of bed in the morning, 10 percent higher than normal?

2. Has your body weight, taken after voiding but before eating or drinking in the morning, dropped 3 percent below normal or more than one or two pounds in one week? Keep in mind that your level of hunger may vary depending on how your body reacts to exercise. Sometimes people feel more hungry when they start a regular aerobics program and sometimes people feel less hungry. Be sure to eat three well-balanced meals that include carbohydrates, protein, and fat.

3. Was the number of hours you slept last night 10 percent fewer than normal?

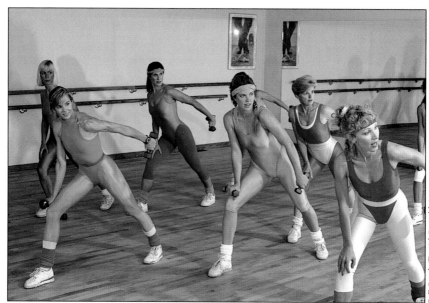

If you answer "no" to all of the questions, feel free to work out at the level you've planned for that day. If you answer "yes" to one of the questions, plan to cut your workout short. If you answer "yes" to two of the questions, be prepared to work out at a lower intensity level. If you answer "yes" to all of the questions, take the day off.

Choosing Your Workouts

The intensity, level, and duration of the workouts that are best for you depend on your present level of conditioning. Your Relative Fitness Level score from chapter 3 will help you determine where to start.

- If you're new to aerobics or if your Relative Fitness Level score was low or below average, you'll probably feel most comfortable doing workouts from the Green and Blue zones. If you plan to follow the sample programs, start with the beginning/easy samples. If you've never done aerobics, be sure you can complete the Green workouts comfortably before you attempt to follow the beginning sample programs. If you're overweight and wish to burn more calories, exercise at low intensity and increase duration with the Blue zone workouts. Be willing to vary your workout intensity to avoid boredom.

- If you have done some aerobics in the past or if your Relative Fitness Level score was average, you'll probably be able to take most of your workouts from the Purple and Yellow zones, and you'll enjoy an occasional harder Orange workout. If you're following the sample programs, you should be able to handle the frequent/moderate samples.

- If you were doing aerobics regularly before picking up this book or if your Relative Fitness Level score was above average or high, you'll be able to take more of your workouts from the high intensity Orange and Red zones. In practice, you'll probably find yourself doing a little bit of everything—mixing in moderate Purple and Yellow workouts as well as low intensity Green and Blue workouts to give yourself a rest after really hard efforts.

The suggested workouts in chapter 13 are based on three-week cycles. Your body will change and adapt to your workouts in only three weeks, so if your goal is health and fitness improvement, you'll need to change your program every three to four weeks, gradually increasing duration, then intensity.

If you choose to deviate from the sample programs, follow these guidelines:

- Let your performance level determine how much, how often, and how hard you work. If you're a beginner, you should train a maximum of three to four times per week. Most of your workouts should come from the Blue and Green zones, but you may want to add some variety (and slightly more intensity) with one workout per week from the Purple zone. If you fall into the moderate category, you can probably handle four to five workouts per week, with most of your workouts coming from the Purple or Yellow zones. If you want to work a little harder, complete one workout per week from the Orange zone. If you're advanced, you should consider five or six workouts per week, and you may want to include as many as two high intensity Orange or Red zone workouts each week.

- Listen to your body. You'll soon be able to judge how it is adapting to each workout. Aerobics is similar to running or weight lifting. Some days you'll feel as if you can push yourself very hard. Other days you may feel very weak. This fluctuation is normal as your body adapts to a regular aerobics program.

- Remember that the higher the number a workout has within a particular zone, the greater the intensity and complexity of that workout. Choose your workouts wisely.

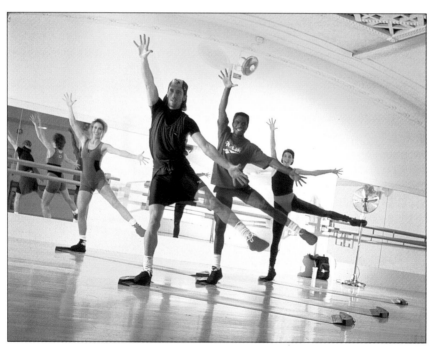

Courtesy of AVIA

- If your goal is to improve your level of health and fitness, you'll need to focus on your workout intensity, duration, and frequency. Studies prove that if your goal is to improve your cholesterol level, reduce risk of heart disease, or metabolize fat, then longer workouts that expend at least 300 calories are recommended. Also, more frequent aerobics sessions per week will help to improve your fitness level.

- Let your body recover. Don't work at a very high intensity and for a long duration two days in a row. Schedule a day of rest or an easy workout (Green or Blue zones), even though you may be an intense aerobics enthusiast. Recovery is essential so you can push harder on your highest intensity and longest duration workout days.

- Vary your aerobics program intensity and types of aerobics workouts as shown in the sample programs. Alternate higher intensity workouts with lower intensity workouts, and vary the types of aerobics workouts you do. This will keep aerobics fun.

Now that you're familiar with a few of the principles on which the sample programs are built, and you have an idea of where you fit, let's take a look at the sample programs.

13

Sample Aerobics Programs

This chapter includes seven different sample training programs, incorporating all forms of aerobics. The programs are merely suggested, based on your present level of conditioning and your fitness goals. Feel free to modify them if the types of workouts are not your preferences. The most important thing for you to remember if you want to see improvement is to stick to a program, whether it's one of these or your own. Consistency is essential.

In the sample workout schedules that follow, the color of the squares indicates the workout zone. The specific workout is denoted by the number inside the square.

Beginning/Easy Aerobics Programs

Beginning does not mean "weak." Beginning levels of intensity are appropriate for all people, of all ages, and all fitness levels. If you're a true beginner, you probably work out for aerobic benefits, weight control, stress management, or for other similar reasons. If you have not done aerobics before, make sure you can comfortably complete each workout in the Green zone before you attempt to follow the beginning schedule.

The three-week schedules that follow should improve your aerobics performance and gradually increase your ability to complete longer and more intense workouts. Three to four workouts are done in a week, with varied durations, intensities, and movement styles (e.g., chair aerobics, LIA, step, or hi/lo). At least one medium intensity, short duration (Purple zone) workout is completed each week.

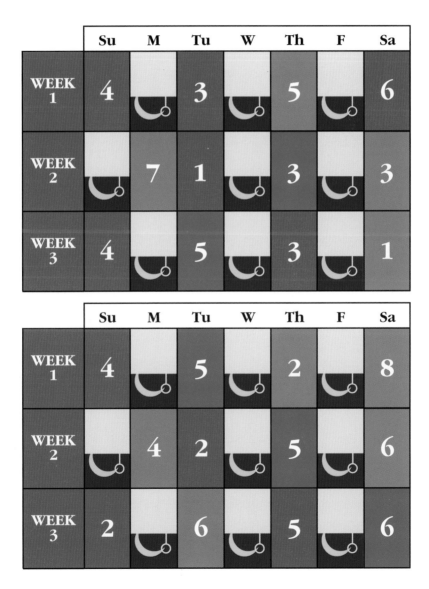

Frequent/Moderate Aerobics Programs

A frequent aerobics enthusiast trains a little longer, faster, harder, and more often than a beginner. It is the next step beyond basic exercising.

Frequent aerobics enthusiasts find excitement in doing more than minimal amounts. They start to explore other movement opportunities and intensities. The schedules offer four to five workouts per week, with varied workout durations, intensities, and movement styles (e.g., step, LIA, HIA, interval, chair aerobics, etc.). Medium intensity, long duration (Yellow zone) workouts are offered at least once each week.

	Su	M	Tu	W	Th	F	Sa
WEEK 1	3		6		1	3	
WEEK 2	2	3	2		4		4
WEEK 3	5		2	6		4	3

	Su	M	Tu	W	Th	F	Sa
WEEK 1	4		7		2	5	
WEEK 2	2	3	2		6		3
WEEK 3	6		3	5		4	6

Competitive/Intense Aerobics Programs

Here you're competing with yourself and your previous workout duration and intensity. Even though you're not competing against anyone else, your objective is to set personal goals for physical and psychological improvement.

If you enjoy these intense workouts, you may consider teaching aerobics classes to aerobics enthusiasts of all levels. Or consider competing in local, regional, national, and international aerobics competitions sanctioned by the National Aerobic Championship (NAC) or the United States Competitive Aerobic Federation (USCAF). Either of these options will require additional training and skills. Mastering the intense workouts will help you determine if you'd like to pursue this next step in the fitness industry.

These programs offer six workouts per week, with varied workout intensities, durations, and movement styles (LIA, hi/lo, interval, step, and slide). Intense workouts are offered once or twice per week. This means that your workout will reach into the high intensity Orange and Red workout zones. The remaining workouts are low or medium intensity. Occasionally, you may have two workouts to choose from on a particular day. I indicate this with a split on the chart. Red workout 5 or 6 is shown 5/6, for example. Choose the aerobics movement style you prefer.

	Su	M	Tu	W	Th	F	Sa
WEEK 1	6	5	7	2	2	7	☾
WEEK 2	4	5	☾	6	5	2	3
WEEK 3	7	☾	2	3	8	5	5

	Su	M	Tu	W	Th	F	Sa
WEEK 1	4/5	3	4	3	4	8	(rest)
WEEK 2	4	2	(rest)	6/7	4	6	5
WEEK 3	8	(rest)	4	4	6	1	6/7

	Su	M	Tu	W	Th	F	Sa
WEEK 1	5	3	4	1	3	6	(rest)
WEEK 2	3	5	(rest)	6	6	1	2
WEEK 3	7	(rest)	2	2	5	5	4/7

The days listed as rest days do not require total inactivity. You may prefer to cross train on these days. Cross training incorporates different forms of fitness sports and activities. For example, walking, biking, swimming, tennis, or running are all great ways to cross train to keep fitness fun. Cross training adds variety, keeps your fitness program exciting, and prevents injury so you can continue to make improvements in your aerobics program.

14

Charting Your Progress

Although aerobics does not have a finish line or require a stopwatch, you can measure improvement and chart progress. Improvement can be measured four ways. Your resting heart rate, your body weight, your percent body fat, and how you feel will each give you insight into how you're doing.

Your heart rate should be taken every morning before you first step out of bed. The lowering of your resting heart rate means that your cardiopulmonary system is improving.

Record your body weight once a week. Step on the scale when you first wake up, after you void, and before you eat or drink anything. Most aerobics enthusiasts choose aerobics for its weight loss benefits, but be careful not to become obsessed with your body weight. It's not necessary to weigh yourself every day. If you are interested in permanent weight loss, only a one- or two-pound loss per week is best. (If you want to take weight off permanently, you need to follow a balanced nutritional program in addition to your aerobics.) Remember that weight loss may not be fat loss. You may also lose muscle mass and fluids. Sudden weight loss of three pounds or more is a sign that you've exceeded optimum training and you need to take a break.

Your percent body fat can be determined by a tape measure or measured by a fitness professional using a skinfold caliper. If you prefer to use a tape measure, follow the guidelines below. Your circumference should decrease over time. You may have access to a fitness professional who can do percent body fat measurements with a skinfold caliper. The average subcutaneous (under the skin) body fat will decrease over time with a consistent aerobics program. Measuring percent body fat is a good way to accurately determine fat losses.

SITES FOR MEASURING THE GIRTH OF CERTAIN BODY PARTS

Chest—at the nipple level

Waist—at the minimal abdominal girth below the rib cage and just above the top of the hip bone

Hips—with feet together, at the level of the symphysis pubis in front and around the maximal protrusion of the buttocks in back

Thigh—at the crotch level and just below the fold of the buttocks

Calf—at the maximum circumference

Ankle—at the minimum circumference, usually just above the ankle bones

Wrist—at the minimum circumference, with arm extended, palm up

RECOMMENDED GIRTH PROPORTIONS FOR WOMEN

Bust—same as the hips

Waist—10 inches less than the bust or hips

Hips—same as the bust

Thighs—6 inches less than the waist

Calves—6 to 7 inches less than the thigh

Ankles—5 to 6 inches less than the calf

Upper Arm—twice the size of the wrist

RECOMMENDED GIRTH PROPORTIONS FOR MEN

Chest—same as the hips

Waist—5 to 7 inches less than the chest or hips

Hips—same as the chest

Thighs—8 to 10 inches less than the waist

Calves—7 to 8 inches less than the thigh

Adapted, by permission, from B. Getchell, 1992, *Physical fitness: A way of life*, 4th ed. (New York: Macmillan Publishing Company), 66.

The last way to measure progress is by your perceived level of intensity and exertion. You should feel good all over during your workouts and you should feel energized after your workouts. If the intensity feels light or easy, it doesn't mean you're not deriving aerobic benefits. If you feel physically challenged, listen to your body's signals to determine if you're working too hard. After a few weeks of aerobics, you should feel physically able to work a little harder.

In addition, your skill level should improve. After a three-week period of aerobics, you should not feel any soreness or stiffness. You'll feel much more comfortable performing all types of movements. You may find yourself moving your entire body with more energy. You'll bend your knees more with the step touch or press your arms higher with the press up. Complex choreography will be easier to do. You may even find yourself wanting to work out longer and with more complex moves. You should feel good about this process because your body and mind have adapted and you have moved to a new skill level of aerobics.

Evaluate your performance by taking the STEP Fit Test every 9 to 12 weeks. Your relative fitness level should improve. If you do not see improvement, you need to reassess your entire aerobics schedule. Remember, consistency is the key to improvement.

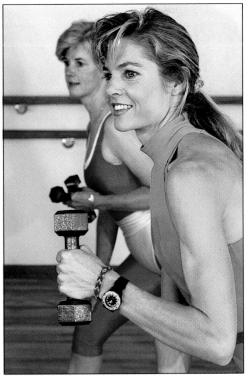

© F-Stock/David Stoecklein

Change does not come easily or instantly. Your body will slowly adapt to your program. A long time from now you'll look back and be proud of how far you've progressed. You'll need to keep accurate records so you can visibly see your progress. I recommend that you keep a diary, journal, or log of your workouts so you can measure your current fitness level and compare it with previous levels.

Use the training log on page 147 to chart your progress. Record the date, your resting heart rate, your workout zone and number, music you used, and comments on how you felt during and after your workout. Summarize your overall feelings about your workout. For example, did you feel tired or energized? Was the workout too easy or too hard? Keep your training log so you have a record of your progress, especially as you do more intense workouts. The more information you record, the easier it will be to evaluate and measure progress.

Commitment is important. If you stop your program for a period of time, you will lose some of the benefits you've gained. You can revert to your original relative fitness level in only two short weeks of inactivity. But if you work out regularly, you'll find that if you do stop for a period of time, returning to your program should not seem too difficult.

I hope your main goal is to incorporate your aerobics program into your lifestyle, making it an activity that you routinely perform. Feel good about getting hooked on the wonderful aerobic benefits, especially the fun of having so much variety in your workouts. Notice how well your clothes fit, how calmly you react to situations at work and at home, and how healthy your whole body feels. You can dramatically improve the quality of your life—and maintain it—if you commit to getting fit and staying fit for the rest of your life.

Date	Pulse / Weight	Workout zone and #	Music	Comments
Su				
M				
Tu				
W				
Th				
F				
Sa				

Summary _____

_____

_____

_____

Aerobics Moves

Arm Movements

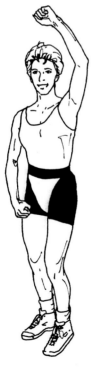

Monkey

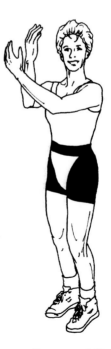

Open and Cross

Arm Movements *(continued)*

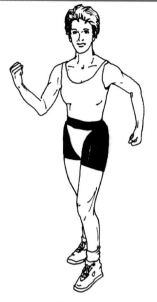

Pump

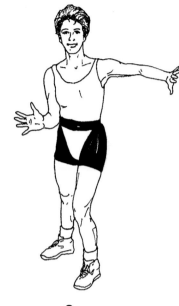

Sway

Chair Aerobics

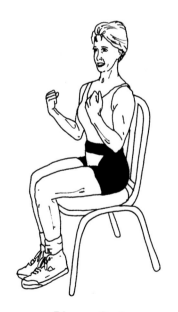

Biceps Curl

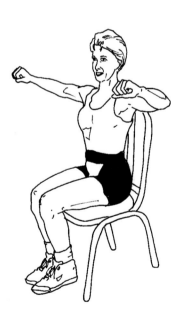

Lateral Deltoid Raise

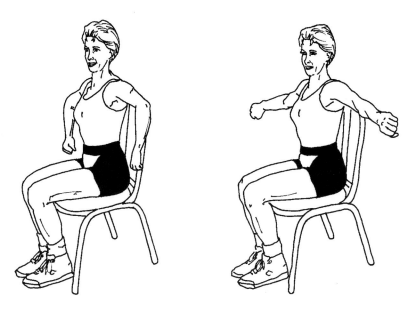

Lateral Triceps Press

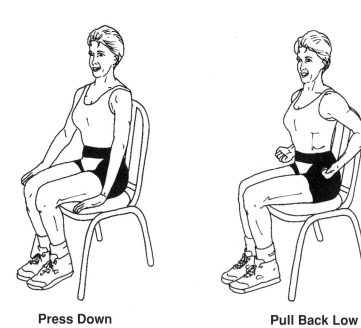

Press Down   **Pull Back Low**

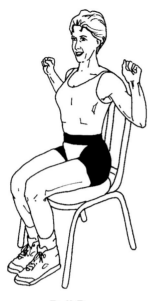

Pull Down

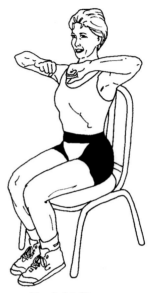

Upright Row

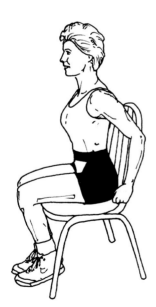

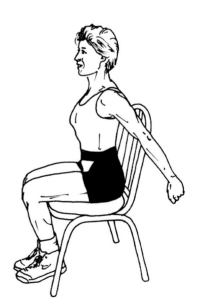

Triceps Kickback

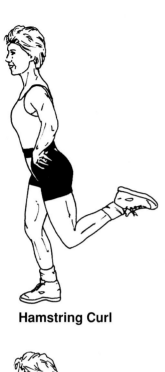

Hamstring Curl

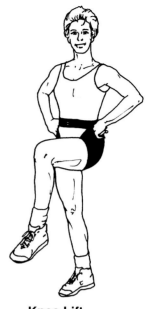

Knee Lift

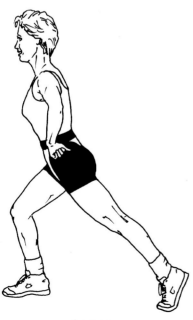

Lunge

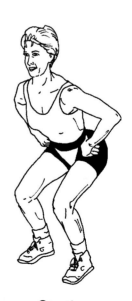

Squat

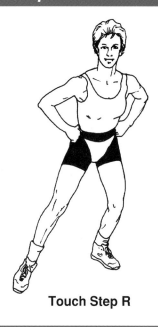

Touch Step R

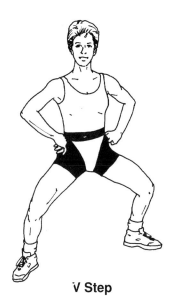

V Step

Moderate Impact Aerobics

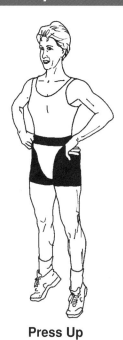

Press Up

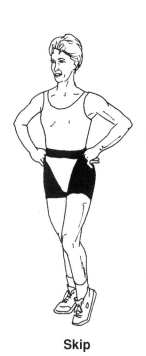

Skip

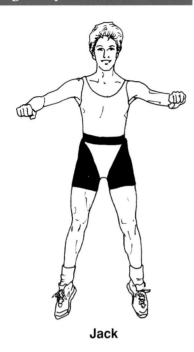

Jack

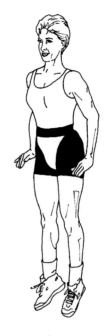

Jump

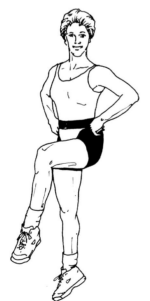

Knee Lift

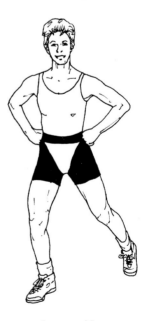

Lunge Hop

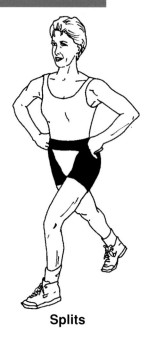

Splits

Step Aerobics

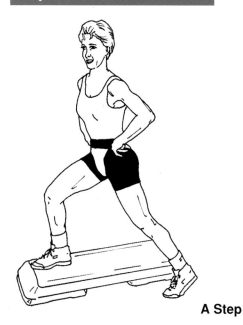
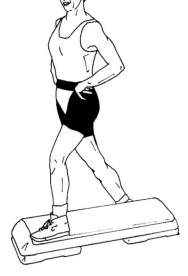

A Step

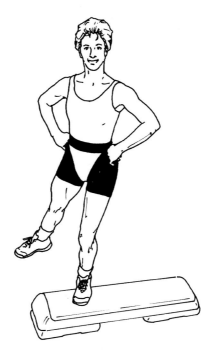

Abductor Lift

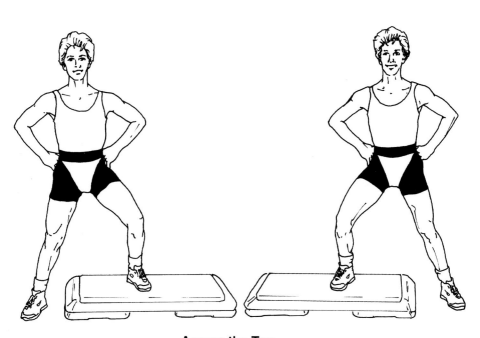

Across the Top

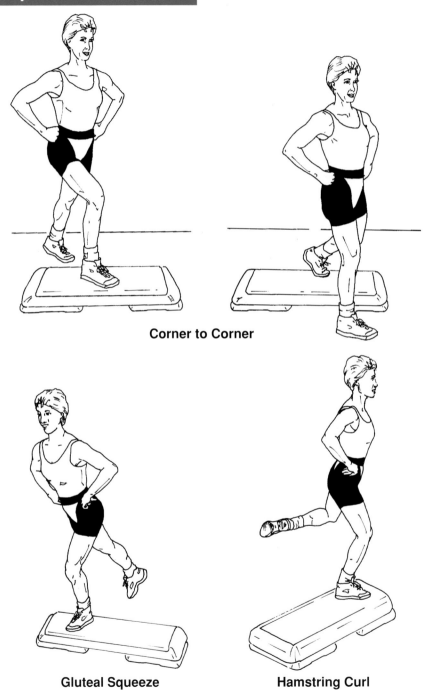

Corner to Corner

Gluteal Squeeze

Hamstring Curl

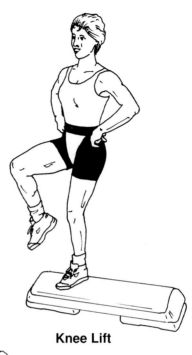

Knee Lift

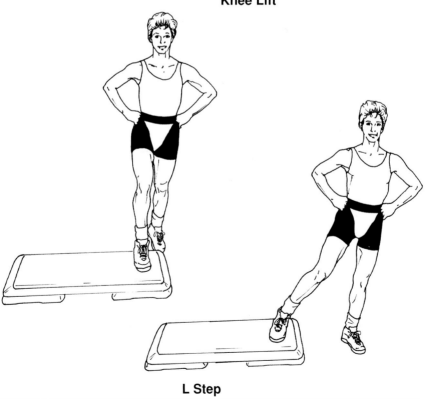

L Step

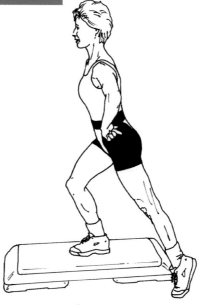

Lunge

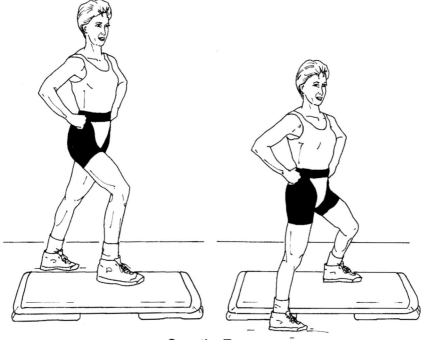

Over the Top

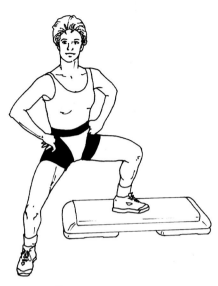

Squat

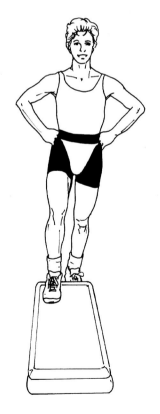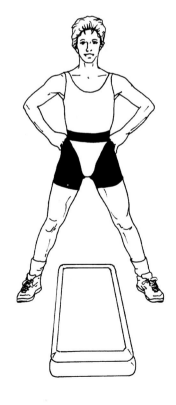

T Step

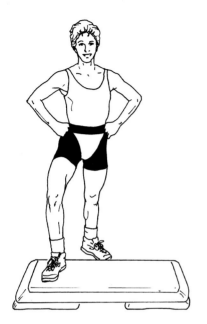 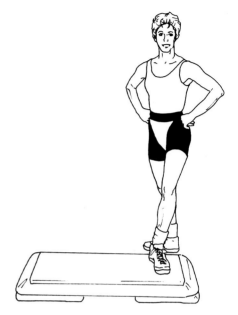

Turn Step

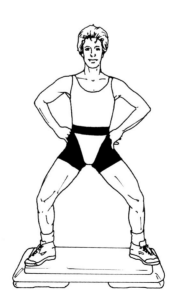

V Step

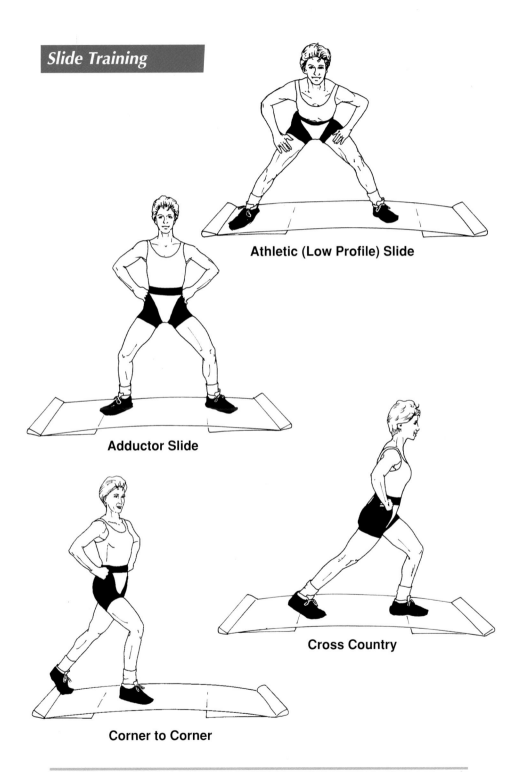

Slide Training

Athletic (Low Profile) Slide

Adductor Slide

Cross Country

Corner to Corner

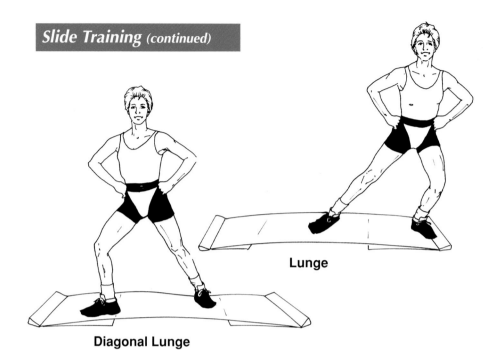

Lunge

Diagonal Lunge

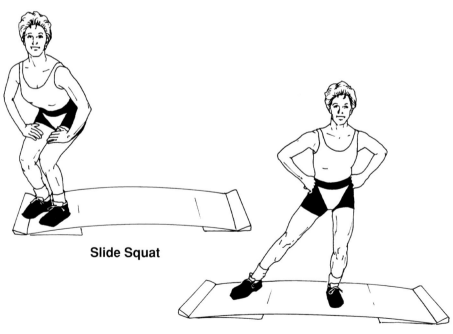

Slide Squat

Stationary Skating Slide

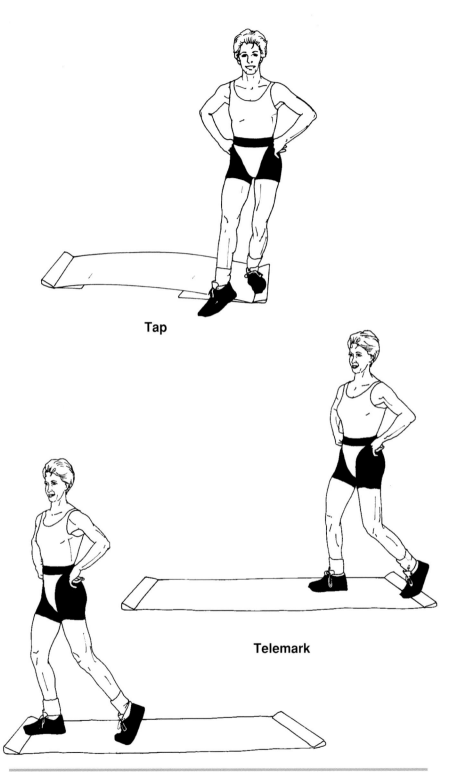

Tap

Telemark

Appendix B

Aerobics Music

You can obtain the music selections used in the workouts on audiocassette from the following companies. This is just a sampling of available music—call Power Productions or Muscle Mixes for up-to-date selections.

Power Productions
1-800-777-BEAT or
801-975-9393

Aerobics Power Mix #18
Aerobics Power Mix #19
Aerobics Power Mix #20
Best of Step, Volume 1
Broadway Power Mix
Broadway Step
Cardio Country
Cardio Country 2
Cardio Power Mix 1
Cardio Power Mix 2
Classic Rock Workout
Club Trax 1
Club Trax 2, Techno Workout

Club Trax 5, Tribal Beats
Club Trax 6, Happy House Workout
Hip Hop Funk
Latin Power Mix
Lynne Brick Power Mix
Mid-Tempo Mix 1
Mid-Tempo Power Mix 1
Mid-Tempo Power Mix 2
Motown Step
Motown Step 2
Power Toning
70's Workout
Step Power Mix
Step Power Mix #6
Step Power Mix #8
Step Power Mix #9

Muscle Mixes Music, Inc.
1-800-52 MIXES or
407-872-7576
   Adding Horsepower Step
      Reebok #12
   The Assembly Line Step Reebok #6
   Disco Fever 1
   Hi-Impact 19
   Increasing Your RPM's Step
      Reebok #10
   Motown

Musica Caliente
Performance Hi #16
Performance Hi+Lo Impact #12
Performance Hi+Lo Impact #17
Resonant Energy
Resonant Energy Step Reebok #13
Rockin' Aerobics
Slide Reebok
Stay on Track Step Reebok #8
Step Reebok #12
Step Reebok Power Combinations II